ROMAN MEDICINE

ROMAN MEDICINE

AUDREY CRUSE

This book is dedicated to the memory of my late husband, Ken
6th January 1925 - 19th May 2004

First published in 2004 by Tempus Publishing
Reprinted 2006

Reprinted in 2011
The History Press
The Mill, Brimscombe Port
Stroud, Gloucestershire GL5 2QG
www.thehistorypress.co.uk

British Library Cataloguing in Publication Data.
A catalogue record for this book is available from the British Library.

ISBN 978 0 7524 1461 4

Typesetting and origination by Tempus Publishing.
Printed and bound in Great Britain by
Marston Book Services Limited, Didcot

CONTENTS

ACKNOWLEDGEMENTS

I wish to thank Peter Kemmis Betty for bringing out a second edition of this book. Amongst other improvements, I have taken the opportunity to correct a few of the 'false certainties' found in the first edition, which were most kindly pointed out to me. Indeed, I am grateful for all the constructive comments which appeared in various reviews of the book and I have acted upon these as far as was possible. Furthermore, I have compiled a new index. My most heartfelt thanks, are due to Laura Perehinec, who has been an extremely helpful editor.

When writing the book, I profited greatly from the works of others and their names are enshrined in the bibliography. I also received help, advice and many kindnesses during the time of the writing and publication of the book in 2004, and I remain greatly indebted to all those friends and colleagues who are acknowledged therein.

This third reprint gives me the opportunity to extend long overdue thanks, first to David Gilbert for his assistance from the very beginning in 1999, when I first received my contract from Tempus and then for his photograph of the hospital at Housesteads Roman Fort on Hadrians' Wall. Second many thanks to Patty Baker, Martin Henig, Ralph Jackson, Helen King and Grahame Soffe who have always been readily available with ideas and information. Third, I am grateful for the encouragement and support that I have received from my husband, Douglas Talintyre. Finally I thank my editors, Tracey Moore and Rowena Williams for their assistance throughout the working of this reprint.

INTRODUCTION

Injury and disease has afflicted the human race since earliest times. Although when unwell many animals instinctively know how to make themselves feel better, the search by human beings for knowledge of their illnesses, of ways to cure and prevent them and for an understanding of their bodily processes, was as much an imperative in the past as it is today. This search defines what medicine is. But medicine is more than this. According to Hippocrates (c.460-370 BC) medicine is an art,[1] and 'the medical colossus of the Roman era,'[2] Galen (c.AD 129-216?), insisted that the good doctor is a philosopher. Medicine is also a skill in that it is the result of practice and knowledge, particularly knowledge of science; thus science is an intrinsic part.

Medicine, therefore, is concerned with the prevention of disease and the art and science of healing. It is as ancient as the human race itself. Healing and bodily health are brought about by the search for, and the application of, remedial substances and the regulation of diet and personal habits. Medicine has only recently been confined to professional, regulated bodies. Today it is a subject of high importance in the politics of church and state; art and philosophy have been translated into medical ethics.

Medicine changes through time. Although basic similarities remain, in many ways ancient medicine bears no resemblance to its modern counterpart. The purpose of this book is to attempt to explain how medicine was practised in the Roman world, to seek out Roman medicine as it was, not how we would like it to have been, nor how close it came to the medicine of today. Neither is the book about 'how nearly they got it right', by comparisons with the familiar concepts and practices of modern medicine, which today are presumed to be the proper way to practise human healing. Every 'medicine' is particular to the culture, time and place in which it finds itself.

Western medicine has a historical pedigree which reaches back to the times of Homeric epic, in which disease and war-wounds are described and treated by divine will or magical incantations, or with surgery or drugs. The *Iliad* and the *Odyssey*, attributed to Homer, were transmitted by ancient oral tradition from the end of the Trojan war, at the beginning of the twelfth century BC, and written down around the eighth century. This is where the name of the paramount god of Greek medicine, Asclepius, is first found, although at this time he was not yet deified. His chief attribute, the snake, is the symbol of medical associations in Britain and abroad, while the sons of Asclepius, Machaon and Podalirius, healers also mentioned in the *Iliad*, are featured today in the arms of the Royal College of Surgeons in London.[3]

Most particularly, Western medicine is indebted to the origins of natural scientific thought in archaic and classical Greece. Hippocrates was a Greek physician born on the island of Cos and known as the 'Father of Medicine'. Many medical treatises are collected under his name, but few, in fact, are his work. Between the seventh and fourth centuries BC, argument and debate concerning different subjects gave rise to the formulation of a variety of competing theories. Questions were asked concerning the identification of individual elements making up the human body and the cosmos, such as earth, air, fire and water. Atomic theory has its roots in this early period. Democritus (*c.*460 BC) thought that all things in the universe were made up of a flux of atoms in a void. Plato (427-347 BC) and his pupil Aristotle (384-322 BC) were concerned with enquiries surrounding the relationship between the body and the soul. Plato taught that the soul (mind or psyche) was immortal and independent of the body and, because the body could influence the mind, one of the duties of the doctor was to teach virtue.

Through Plato the tradition evolved in Western thought whereby an important part of medicine consisted of understanding human nature, or the psyche. Good health depended on temperance and wisdom, on self-control achieved through moderation in the consumption of food and wine, and in sex and physical exercise. Thinking good thoughts led to *sophrosyne*, soundness of mind.[4] Aristotle also investigated the natural world and was interested in explanations concerning anatomy and physiology. He used findings from animal dissections in his research, although he did not distinguish between veins and arteries.

Thinking good thoughts was also required of those who entered the temples of Asclepius. Throughout this period, religious medicine was an important part of life. Healer deities resided at cult centres, such as those erected for Asclepius at Epidaurus, Cos or Pergamum. Here the sick would sleep in order to experience healing dreams. Another important healer-deity was Amphiaraus, found at Oropus near Boeotia. He fulfilled a similar function. However, such cult centres cannot be regarded as early types of a 'hospital' because the sick were not given any form of continuous therapy, nursing care or food. Another aspect of religious medicine to take place at cult centres was pilgrimage. Gifts, often including animals, (*1*) first-fruits, garments and anatomical models of parts of the body, would be carried to the deity, as

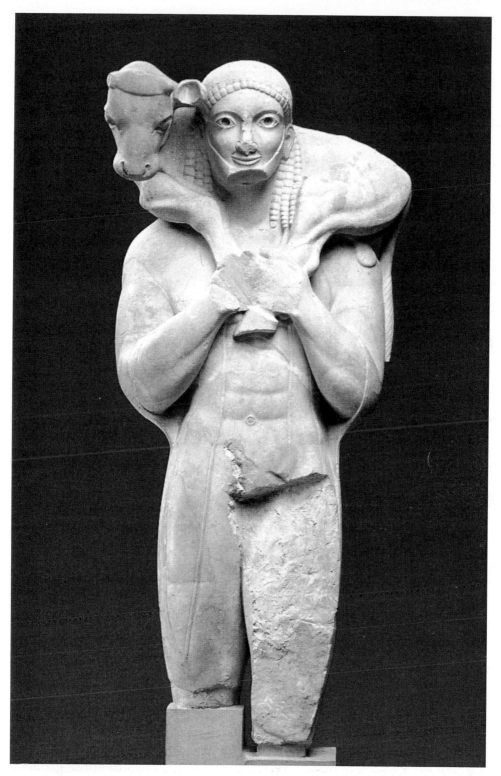

1 The Calf-Bearer, *c.*575–550 BC. *From the Acropolis Museum, Athens*

a request either for healing or for fecundity for themselves, their animals or their crops.

Hospitals were a natural outcome of Rome's military policy. As the Empire expanded its frontiers into distant and hostile territories, suitable places where the sick and wounded could rest and be cared for were needed. Although little is known about its foundation, the Roman military medical provision evolved from this need and hospitals, *valetudinaria*, were provided in forts and fortresses. Greek doctors, including Claudius' personal physician, Caius Stertinius Xenophon of Cos, Scribonius Largus (*c*.AD 1-50) from Sicily, and Dioscorides (*fl. c*.AD 40-90) of Anazarbus, in Roman Cilicia (who may have come to Britain with Claudius' invasion force), were among the army medical personnel.

The distinction between veins and arteries, although not discovered by Aristotle when in Athens, may have been realised at other centres of study. Some of these have already been mentioned above. Many theories came from Praxagoras of Cos (*c*.340 BC) and Diocles of Carystus (*c*.320 BC) in Euboea. Later, in the second century AD, Galen decided that blood was made in the liver where it became mixed with foods in the form of chyle. This nourishment for the extremities was carried by veins which also originated in the liver. According to Galen, arteries commenced in the heart, although full understanding of blood circulation was not to come until much later, with the work of William Harvey, published in 1628.

In 331 BC, Alexander the Great, whose tutor had been Aristotle, founded the city of Alexandria, ushering in the Hellenistic period. When Alexander died in 323, Egypt was ruled by a line of Macedonian kings, the Ptolemies, and a royal dynasty was established. The city of Alexandria became very wealthy. The library and museum were founded and a great international centre of study and research grew up. It continued at least into the second century AD and possibly lasted throughout the Roman period in Egypt (30 BC-*c*. AD 323). Galen is known to have studied at Alexandria, where one of the most important subjects to be researched was anatomy. According to Celsus (*De Med*. pref. 23-6) human dissection was performed. Two of the foremost medical scientists to travel to the great city were Erasistratus of Ceos (330-255 BC) and Herophilus of Chalcedon (*c*.330-260 BC). New discoveries were made in anatomy and physiology and, following the ideas of Alcmaeon of Croton and Diogenes of Apollonia, the brain and not the heart was found to be the seat of intellectual activity.

Among other subjects to be researched in the new city were pharmacology and botany. In the reign of Augustus, after his conquest of Egypt in 31 BC, strange and new ingredients became incorporated into the Roman pharmacopoeia. Later, the expansion of the Empire all round the Mediterranean basin, beyond the Euphrates to Asia, further increased the range of medicinal drugs that could be available. Three routes lay open to a rich diversity of plant-life in the Far East. First by the Black Sea, through the Oxus and by northern Bactria (modern Afghanistan, Tadzhikistan and Kirghizstan); secondly, from Syria down the Euphrates to Nisa and across Persia; finally, the route through the Red Sea and the Indian Ocean.[5]

In the later Empire, after the conversion to Christianity of the Emperor Constantine, the cult of Asclepius was supplanted by Christianity and the first non-military houses where the sick could be cared for were established in the Greek East. Literary and epigraphic sources refer to these as *xenodocheia* and *nosokomeia*. One of the first to be built was that of the bishop St Basil of Caesarea. He provided physicians, nurses, rehabilitation and after-care in his *ptocheion*. This was technically 'a house for the poor', although it was also used for sufferers from other misfortunes, including disease. According to St Jerome, the first hospital in the West was founded in Rome by a wealthy Christian widow, Fabiola, in around AD 350.

Plagues cause social upheaval and change. The chronological framework of the book is bounded by the three most devastating pestilences, known from literary sources, to have occurred in the ancient world. First, the plague in Athens (430-426 BC) which brought about the end of the Athenian Empire; secondly, the 'Antonine Plague', brought back to the Roman Empire by troops returning from campaigns in the Near East. This plague raged for fifteen years and claimed the lives of two emperors. Lastly, in late antiquity, *c.*AD 542, the plague of Justinian lasted for more than fifty years. Recorded by Procopius, the Greek historian, it may have been one of the factors that contributed to the ultimate failure of Justinian's schemes for reviving the Roman Empire.

It is generally accepted that 'rational medicine' describes the type of medical practice which looks for the cause of a disease before prescribing its treatment and 'irrational' describes magic and superstition. However, when viewed alongside the manifest deficiencies of early healing systems, it is possible to construe the use of magic as 'rational'. The question rests on an attitude of respect regarding the beliefs of other peoples. These are aptly juxtaposed by King when she writes[6] that 'the Greeks believed in the wandering womb, whilst we believe in hormones'. 'Scientific', although used to describe the work of the 'natural scientists' and Hippocratic and Galenic medicine, is better used when applied to modern medicine. Finally, 'classical' is used to describe the medicine of the classical period, which embraces most of the fifth and fourth centuries BC.

To conclude, Roman medicine did not arise out of a vacuum, neither is it a single discipline that can be neatly packaged into a linear narrative. On the contrary, Roman medicine is a complex and wide-ranging subject. Its research involves not only older systems of medicine, such as those of the archaic (before 500 BC), classical (500-300 BC), and hellenistic (after 300 BC) periods of the Greek world, but also many of the different cultures which became incorporated into the Roman Empire. These include the medicine of

Ancient Egypt, particularly that of the Graeco-Roman period, during which the centre at Alexandria flourished. In Italy, Roman medicine incorporated Etruscan technical achievements and certain aspects of Etruscan magico-religious healing. Following discussions of these, many of the brief references included in this introduction will be expanded upon, and Roman medicine, as practised during the Roman Republic and Empire, will be discussed in more detail. Sources available are archaeological, for example skeletal evidence, anatomical votive objects and finely-made surgical instruments. Sources are also architectural, in the form of buildings such as baths, aqueducts, sewers and traces of possible military hospitals. Evidence for herbal remedies is discussed, in addition to epigraphy and documentary and literary sources.

GREEK CULT AND MEDICINE

In the ancient Greek world religion was based on myths and legends which reached back into earliest times. Some myths were already ancient before dramatists such as Aeschylus, Sophocles, Euripides and Aristophanes reworked the old stories as drama in order to reflect contemporary issues and as vehicles for their art. Myths embody truths, differing mythologies demonstrate the possibility for more than one single view on a question. For the Greeks and Romans, myths and legends were traditional ways of explaining the mysteries of life and the uncontrollable forces of Nature.

Although Greek myth supposes that diseases were absent at the moment of creation, no time is lost in introducing Pandora and her dowry to the human race. Several myths reflect contemporary ideas about the beginnings of Greek medicine and the origins of disease. The poet Hesiod (c.late eighth century BC) describes the ills that await men and women in times to come. 'Sicknesses visit men by day, and others by night, uninvited, bringing ills to mortals, silently…'. Hesiod also tells of the myth of Pandora who, on opening her jar, 'let loose harsh toils and grim sickness upon mankind'.[1] Nevertheless, 'Hope' was allowed to remain clinging under the lid, allowing for the development of medical enquiry. The poet Aeschylus (fl. 525-456 BC), in his play *Prometheus Bound* uses a myth which tells how Prometheus gave man medicine: 'I showed them how to mix mild healing herbs / and so protect themselves against all maladies'.[2] Another myth which attempts to account for the origins of herbal medicine is that of Cheiron the centaur in Homer. Such myths, reflecting the anxieties of ancient peoples concerning disease, disability and misfortune, were already ancient when used by early writers.

The earliest evidence for the practice of medicine in ancient Greece is met in prehistory with the Mycenaeans, whose proficiency in the skills of healing is attested archaeologically on settlement sites and in tombs. The use of opium, known mainly from ritual, is seen in the Gazi goddess[3] (*colour plate 1*), dating from 1350–1250 BC, into whose diadem-headdress are tucked stalks of poppy-seed heads; coincidentally, according to tradition, this is the time of the Trojan wars.[4] Moreover, the Homeric poems, which tell the story of those wars, and which also emerged in prehistory, bear witness to the care of the sick and wounded, many of whom were treated with medicinal herbs either mixed with wine or applied directly to wounds. It is noteworthy that more than sixty plant varieties are named in Homer.[5]

Medicine has an important place in Homer's epic world and reference to disease occurs early, in the plague cast by Apollo on the Greek army at Troy. Apollo, striking from afar, drives 'the foul pestilence along the host and the people perished' (*Iliad* I.10). Apollo was a healing deity and the most important divine supporter of the Trojans. He inflicted the plague upon the Greek army before Troy as punishment for the abduction of Chryseis, daughter of his priest Calchas. Later, after Agamemnon has surrendered the girl, Apollo is appeased. Healed of his anger, he causes the plague to cease. Homer includes a doctor among the following: '…one who works for the people, either / a prophet, or a healer of sickness, or a skilled workman, / or inspired singer, or one who can give delight by his singing'. The idea that healers were 'journeymen' is also shown here (*Odyssey* XVII.383–5). The inclusion of the 'healer of sickness' with community workers and skilled workmen, is the first reference to an important aspect of ancient medicine – that it was regarded as a *techne*, a craft or a skill, comparable to other *technai*, such as the work of a sculptor,[6] or a builder.

Apollo was the father of Asclepius. Although Homer refers to Asclepius only once by name (*Iliad* II.731), his presence in the poem is important, for medicine as taught and practised by him in a later period was certainly not a creation out of nothing. When the Greeks sailed against Troy they invited two heroes, the sons of Asclepius, who were also respected doctors, to join the army. Machaon and Podalirius were pupils of Cheiron the centaur, who was a wise and kind friend (*Iliad* IV.219; XI.831); an unusual thing in a centaur. Asclepius, too, had been a pupil of Cheiron.

As an inspired singer, the healer could use an incantation (*epode*) as an haemostatic, like the sons of Autolycus (*Odyssey* XIX.457–458):

> The dear sons of Autolykos were busy to tend him,
> and understandingly they bound up the wound of stately
> Odysseus, and singing incantations over it
> stayed the black blood,…

Incantation may have been as appropriate in Homer's time as 'music therapy' is today – regarded by some people as questionable, even though many claims have been made for positive results. The poet's narrative is a skilful inter-weaving of realistic detail and the imagined world. Allusions to things medical in Homer vary from realistic descriptions of wounds, attesting a certain degree of understanding of anatomy, to the treatment of these by means of medicinal plants. Although reference is made in only two places to bandaging, this does not necessarily mean a lack of knowledge or use. It could also indicate that the dry scab was well known to be a natural 'bandage'.[7]

Both the *Iliad* and the *Odyssey* speak of fearful injuries suffered in battle, caused by weapons such as arrows, spears, swords, jagged rocks or stones. Homeric heroes know where to strike in order to finish off the enemy quickly. The result of a blow depends more on the region and the organs involved than the weapon used. The descriptions of woundings attest knowledge of the anatomical positions of the major organs and of the most likely consequences of injuries to each. For example, Aeneas is struck by a huge rock on the hip at a place called the cup-socket. The blow 'breaks the two tendons' and crushes the cotyloid socket. Aeneas falls to his knees and faints from the pain. Aphrodite, his mother, Apollo and Artemis all protect him and his cure is so rapid that he returns to fight the same day. (*Iliad* V.297-317; 431-70; 514-18.) Another example where anatomical detail is shown is at the death of Diomedes (*Iliad* XVI.480-1): 'Patroklos... with the brazen spear, the shaft escaping his hand was not flung vainly / but struck where the beating heart is closed in the arch of the muscles'.

Eye conditions were a great concern in the ancient world and the theme of blindness all too frequently occupied the Greek mind (*colour plate 2*). It is used by the Muses in the *Iliad* (II.595-600), when, enraged by his boasts, they desired to punish the Thracian bard, Thamrys when, at the same time, he was deprived of his voice. The gods themselves blinded the Theban seer Tiresias (*Odyssey* X.492-5). On the other hand, the bard Demodocus was blind as a result of the special affection of the Muses, 'She reft him of his eyes, but she gave him the sweet singing art' (*Odyssey* VIII.63-64), perhaps a reference to Homer himself. Blindness could also have been an affliction from birth. In Greek thought, physical blindness could suggest psychic or spiritual insight. In Sophocles' *Oedipus*, King Oedipus is said to 'see better' after he is blinded. Blindness is rationalised as a gift, or a punishment, bestowed by the gods. Such a rationalisation would go a long way towards helping the sufferer to accept the disability.

At the *Iliad* XVI.28 'Healers skilled in medicine are working to cure their wounds', and at the *Iliad* XI.514-5, Homer tells us that 'A healer is a man worth many men in his knowledge / of cutting out arrows and putting kindly medicines on wounds'. The wounded are carried off the battlefield and tended on nearby ships (*Iliad* XI.824-5). After the wounding of Machaon, the first attentions he received were a seat, story-telling and a cup of 'Pramnian wine, and grated goats-milk cheese into it / with a bronze grater, and scattered with her hand white barley into it' (*Iliad* XI.638). Later, Machaon's wound was washed with warm water by the same woman, 'Hekamede the lovely-haired', (*Iliad* XIV.6). The only remedy in Homer for haemorrhage, apart from the dry scab already mentioned, was the *epode* refered to above and the application of a pounded unnamed root (*Iliad* XI.841-7). This may have been an onion, or *achillea* (woundwort) or *aristolochia*, a herb used for the relief of birth-pangs. Moreover, Homer shows much confidence in speaking of medicine when Patroclus is described removing an arrow from the thigh of Machaon:

> Patroklos laid him there and with a knife cut the sharp tearing arrow out of his thigh, and washed the black blood running from it with warm water, and, pounding it up in his hands, laid on a bitter root to make the pain disappear, one which stayed all kinds of pain. And the wound dried, and the flow of blood stopped.

The need for cleanliness was also recognised. It is seen in the use of fire and brimstone, 'the cure of evils... to sulphur the hall', after the slaughter of the suitors (*Odyssey* XXII.480-495). There is also an element of ritual purification here. Odysseus then cleaned his 'palace, house and courtyard alike, with the sulphur'. In some ways the 'ritual cleansing' of the ancient world can be seen as hygiene. We know that certain bacteria are 'polluting', or 'infectious', but for the ancients pollution could come from wrong actions as well as from the physical events of birth, death and sex.[8]

Arrowheads were made of iron or bronze. Some were tricuspids, with three barbs (*Iliad* V.393), but most had two. These were thin enough to break off when pulled through a leather belt (*Iliad* IV.210-19). The damage to human tissue may be easily imagined; 'as they were pulled out the sharp barbs were broken backwards'. Macheon, called to treat Menelaus, 'sucked out the blood and in skill laid healing medicines on it / that Cheiron in friendship long ago had given his father'. One of these arrow-heads was found in Troy VIIa, lying in the rubble in the middle of the street.[9]

Although opium is not mentioned in Homer it would have been easy to come by. Jewellery and clay objects in the shape of opium poppy-heads, like the headdress of the Gazi goddess described above, attest the availability of the drug from Asia Minor to Greece. Sometimes the poppy-heads in these objects are artificially slit, demonstrating the way that the latex could drip out to be collected. Book IV of the *Odyssey* (lines 220-35) finds Helen in Egypt with Menelaos and Telemachos. The conversation turns on sad memories of Troy. Helen, in kindness, casts a medicine into their wine 'of heartsease, free of gall, to make one forget all sorrows'. This was probably opium, for 'in Egypt, the fertile earth produces the greatest number of medicines and every man is a doctor there and more understanding than men elsewhere'; they belong to the race of the healer-god Paion (later identified with Apollo). It was Paion who healed the wound of the violent Aries when he applied a soothing medicine to it (*Iliad* V.900-4), 'since he, Aries, was not one of the mortals'. Thus it is also demonstrated that the Gods require the services of a divine doctor.

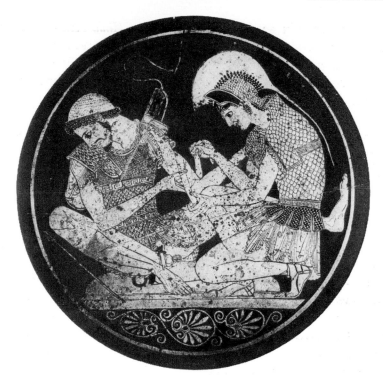

2 Achilles binds the arm of Patroclus

However, the juice of a fig tree, although it could curdle white milk rapidly, as described in the simile in the *Iliad* V.902, has been shown by Majno in his laboratory tests, to actually prevent the clotting of blood.[10]

SOURCES

The value of literary sources has been demonstrated above. However, some Homeric medical scenes are interpreted by iconographical representation on works dating to the Greek and Roman periods. The blinding of the lyre-player, Thamrys, is figured on an Attic hydria of the fifth century BC, seen in the Ashmolean Museum, Oxford (No.530). Therapies practised in the ancient world are also seen in art from both classical Greece and the later Roman period. An illustration by Sosias on a vase of *c.*500 BC depicts Achilles binding the forearm of Patroclus (*2*). Wounds were sometimes treated with iron-scrapings. This is illustrated in a Roman bas-relief from Herculaneum which depicts another scene from the myths of the Trojan wars, in which Achilles applies scrapings from his lance to the injury of Telephus.

In contrast to poetry, which could be more easily remembered and was transmitted verbally through many generations, written prose developed

slowly in the Greek world. Once it appeared, medical writers, historians
and writers of speeches and aphorisms were quick to make use of it. This
happened simultaneously in different areas. Herodotus (*c*.490–*c*.425 BC) was
one of the first to use the new medium. He was also interested in physicians and medicine. Although records were made on stone, writing in ink
on papyrus was predominant by the classical period. Egypt, of course, had
the monopoly on papyrus. Other archaeological sources are also available,
particularly with reference to cult centres.

HEALER–GODS AND THEIR SANCTUARIES

Many sanctuaries in Greece date back at least to Mycenean times and some
continued through the Roman period and beyond. Healing deities occupied
natural sites, ranging from rivers and mountain springs to peak sanctuaries
(*3*). Nymphs of Artemis, according to literary sources, were found in brooks
and streams. They cured, among other maladies, eye diseases. These ideas
were deeply rooted in ancient belief. Apart from Apollo, who possessed
other interests besides that of health, the two best-known powers of healing
in ancient Greece belonged to Apollo's son, Asclepius, and the demi-god
Amphiaraus of Oropus. Although the cult of Asclepius was to spread
throughout the Greek world as far as Cilicia, and then to Rome and the West,
that of Amphiaraus remained centred on his sanctuary at Oropus, situated on
the borders of Attica and Boeotia.

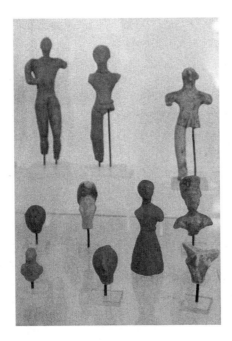

3 Votive figurines from the Middle
Minoan peak sanctury of Prinias, Siteia

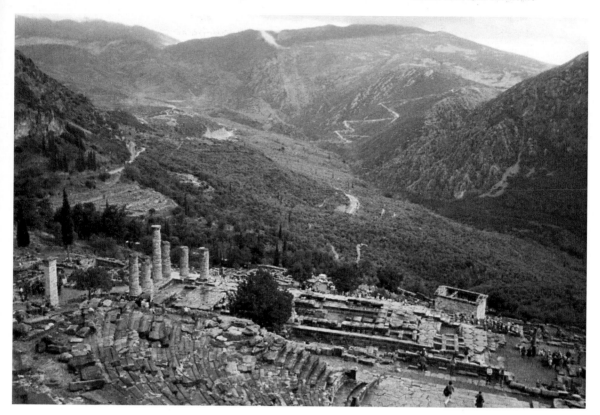

4 The sanctuary of Apollo at Delphi

APOLLO

In Greek mythology Apollo (*colour plate 3*) was twin brother to Artemis. Whilst he was god of the plague and the healing hymn, Artemis was the goddess of childbirth and fertility. The nature of Apollo is complicated. Although he was subject to the human passions of lust and jealousy, this was balanced by testimonies at his shrine at Delphi (*4*) to another aspect of his nature, that of moral excellence. In the fifth century, proverbs engraved on his temple – the method used for the dissemination of wisdom at the time – fully expressed this particular attribute. Among the many epigrams discovered were two which today continue to be regarded as useful: 'nothing in excess' and that other famous Greek injunction, 'first know thyself'. Oracles and healing sanctuaries are often found on the same site; one example is the sanctuary of Amphiaraus of Oropus. However, at Delphi, there is no direct evidence for a healing cult, although Apollo was first and foremost a healing deity and this was his major shrine. In Roman times, Apollo retained his Greek name and other major sanctuaries; for example Delos, also sacred to Apollo, became just as important as Delphi.

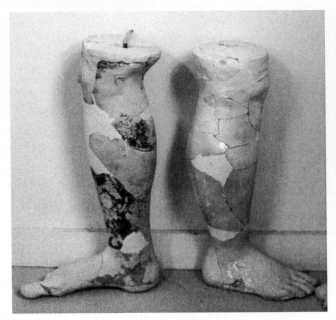
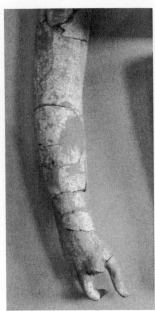

5 Votive limbs from Corinth

ASCLEPIUS

The conception of Asclepius was straightforward. Apollo, seeing Coronis, a mortal nymph and daughter of King Phylegys of Thessaly whilst she was bathing, desired her and seduced her and the violent birth of Asclepius followed in due course. However, before this could happen, her father arranged a marriage with a mortal prince and the god felt slighted. Apollo was told of the marriage arrangements by a raven which at the time possessed white plumage. As a punishment for bearing the bad news Apollo cursed the bird and turned his plumage black (*colour plate 3*). Because of Coronis' forthcoming marriage and her apparent adultery, jealous Apollo tore his unborn son out of her womb and gave the prematurely-born infant for parenting to Cheiron the centaur, by whom he was nurtured and taught the art of medicine on Mount Pelion. Because of his mixed parentage, controversy has always existed as to whether Asclepius (*colour plate 4*) was a god or a hero.

Several myths surround the nativity of Asclepius. They are attempts to account for both his mortality and his divine status. In Homer a few indirect references appear but there is no special mention of his epiphany as in Hesiod and Pindar, where his death caused by Zeus is described. The reason for Zeus' action was that, in answer to a plea from Artemis, Asclepius restored her favourite, Hippolytus son of Theseus, to life. Zeus was further angered when Hades, god of the underworld, complained about the unequal numbers of souls or persons inhabiting the two different worlds, due to the miraculous interventions of

Asclepius. In his anger Zeus slew the healer with a thunderbolt. Later Apollo, son of Zeus, raised Asclepius from the dead and rewarded him with divine status. Asclepius' wife was Epione and their two daughters were Hygea and Panacea; their sons, Podalirius and Machaon, are already referred to above. In art Asclepius is also frequently seen with Telesphorus (*colour plates 5* and *6*), god of convalescence, usually depicted as a small hooded figure, similar in appearance to the so-called *genii cucullati* found in Britain and Gaul. Other sanctuaries belonging to Asclepius, known through texts and archaeological excavation, are found at Athens, Corinth, Piraeus, Pergamum and Cos. An important feature in all those mentioned is the proximity of a theatre. At Corinth, votive limbs from the sanctuary are exhibited in the site museum (*5*).

Originally Asclepius was known as a Thessalian king and a mortal healer. His sons, Podalirius and Machaon, came from Trikka in Thessaly where they already worked as doctors. However, in the *Iliad*, Homer merely refers in passing to the hero Asclepius. It was later, in classical times, that he was deified. He then became the focus for a healing cult in temples through the Greek and Roman world. His serpents were held to be sacred and sometimes assumed the functions of Asclepius himself. Furthermore, in their annual shedding of the old skin and the growing of a new one, snakes were symbols of renewal (*6*, *7* and *8*).[11]

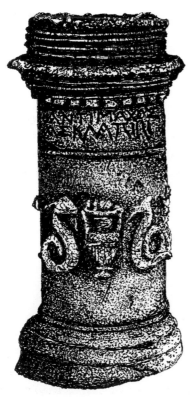

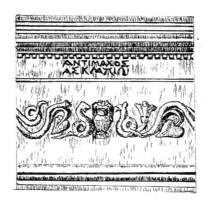

6 Snakes, the chief attribute of Aesclepius featured on a stone altar at Butrint, Albania

EPIDAURUS: THE ARCHAEOLOGY

Epidaurus was the first and most important shrine of Asclepius. The area is known to have been associated with a healing cult since the sixteenth century BC. At first it was the shrine of the hero-deity Malleatus who was god of the hunt, hence the association with hounds. Sometime later this deity was conflated with Apollo who was then known as 'Apollo Malleatus'. His cult was centred on Mount Kynortion which rises above the sacred precinct of Epidaurus (*9*). In Greek, the name reflects the hound epithet.[12] The remains of sacrifices performed during the seventh century BC have been discovered by archaeologists, in addition to vestiges of much later temples and other buildings. These could have been guest-houses for pilgrims visiting the shrine

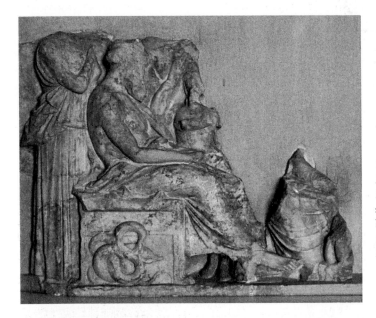

7 Snakes featured on *Left* a) a funerary stelae; *Below* b) a votive plaque showing Hygea standing behind the god. *From the National Archaeological Museum, Athens*

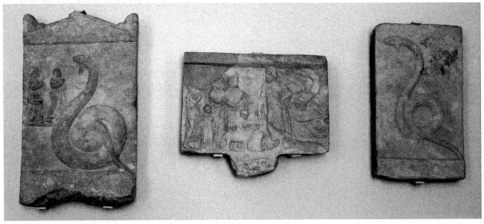

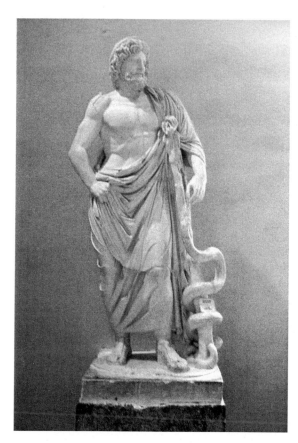

8 Left A statue of Asclepius, from Epidaurus

9 Below Mount Kynortion rises above the sanctuary of Asclepius at Epidaurus; the theatre is in the foreground

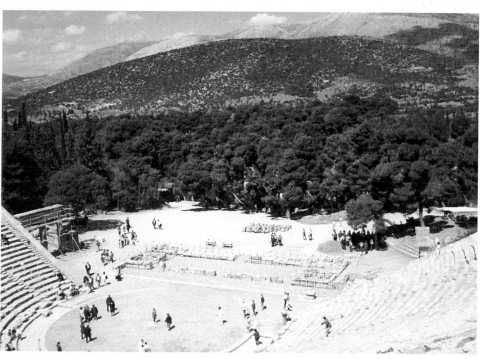

and in many instances the finds confirm that the cult of Asclepius at Epidaurus continued at least until the imperial period.[13]

Writing in the second century AD during and after the reigns of Hadrian and Antoninus Pius, Pausanias, a Greek doctor (according to Levi, 1971) and a travel–writer, was personally devoted to Asclepius. He provides many references to the god concerning his birth and background. In his 'Guide to Greece'[14] Pausanias records statuary and works of art depicting Asclepius, some of which are shown in contemporary or later coinage. He writes of the territory of the Argolid: 'this whole land is especially sacred to Aesculapius',[15] such was his devotion to the god. Pausanias records that the Emperor Antoninus Pius was responsible for many kindnesses here, one of which was, whilst yet a senator, to build a house for women in labour: 'here a man can die and a woman bear her child without sacrilege'[16] (childbirth was regarded as potentially polluting). It is not known exactly when the god arrived at Epidaurus and took over from Apollo but the general opinion is that Apollo was venerated from the seventh century and the cult of Asclepius arrived in the sixth or fifth century.

The site has been under excavation by Greek archaeologists since 1881 until the present time. Buildings within the sanctuary have been located and identified. These include the temples of Asclepius and Artemis, the stadium, hotel (*katagogion*), banqueting hall, baths, gymnasium and tholos (*thymele*). The most complete building is the theatre, a building of great beauty and magnificence; the original *orchestra* remains. The fifty-five tiers of seats are restored and the theatre is used today for the performance of the Greek plays for which it was originally built. A small museum houses many sculptures and artefacts rescued from the site itself. No anatomical votives were found at Epidaurus. Stone slabs, *iamata*, bear inscriptions recording case-histories and cures received by pilgrims to the shrine; four of them were found during excavation and two are virtually intact. Pausanias writes:

> In my day there are six left of the stone tablets standing in the enclosure, though there were more in antiquity. The names of men and women healed by Asclepios are engraved on them, with the diseases and how they were healed.

A few of the cures seen by Pausanias appear below:[17]

> Ambrosia of Athens, blind of one eye. She came as a suppliant to the god. As she walked about in the Temple she laughed at some of the cures as incredible and impossible, that the lame and the blind should be healed by merely seeing a dream. In her sleep she had a vision. It seemed to her that the god stood by her and said he would cure her, but that in payment he would ask her to dedicate to the Temple a silver pig as a memorial of her ignorance. After saying this, he cut

the diseased eyeball and poured in some drug. When day came she walked out sound.

Edelstein, 1945, stele 1-4

Euphanes, a boy of Epidaurus. Suffering from stone he slept in the Temple. It seemed to him that the god stood by him and asked: 'What will you give me if I cure you?' 'Ten dice,' he answered. The god laughed and said to him that he would cure him. When day came he walked out sound.

Edelstein 1945, stele 1-8

A man with an abscess within his abdomen. When asleep in the Temple he saw a dream. It seemed to him that the god ordered the servants who accompanied him to grip him and hold him tightly so that he could cut open his abdomen. The man tried to get away, but they gripped him and bound him to a door knocker. Thereupon Asclepius cut his belly open, removed the abscess, and, after having stitched him up again, released him from his bonds. Whereupon he walked out sound, but the floor of the Abaton was covered with blood.

Edelstein, 1945, stele 11-27

Cleinatas of Thebes with lice. He came with a great number of lice on his body, slept in the Temple, and saw a vision. It seemed to him that the god stripped him and made him stand upright, naked, and with a broom brushed the lice from off his body. When day came he left the Temple well.

Edelstein, 1945, stele 11-28

Gorgias of Heracleia with pus. In a battle he had been wounded by an arrow in the lung and for a year and a half had suppurated so badly that he filled sixty-seven basins with pus. While sleeping in the Temple he saw a vision. It seemed to him the god extracted the arrow point from his lung. When day came he walked out well, holding the point of the arrow in his hands.

Edelstein, 1945, stele 11-30

THE CULT OF ASCLEPIUS

In order to receive healing dreams, it was necessary for the patient to sleep in the *abaton*. Asclepius would appear during the dream to give his instructions. These would be interpreted by specially trained priests. Before approaching the god, the patient was required to follow a prescribed ritual. In the temples of Asclepius this procedure was not at all arduous or unpleasant. Nothing unkind or grasping is found in his ministry. Asclepius charged no entrance fee and made few requests of his patients; he merely required that the suppliant should purify their body by washing and have good thoughts. Many of the testimonies show that the god especially cared for such qualities. He only refused to help those who came to him in dishonesty, or who had a high regard for great personal wealth. Testimonies found both at the temple at Epidaurus and at Lambaesis carried the inscription: 'Pure must the person be who goes inside the fragrant temple, purity means to think nothing but holy thoughts'.[18]

SACRED SLEEP, DREAM ORACLES, INCUBATION, THE ABATON

To prepare for sacred sleep, the patient's mind should be cleared of all worldly thoughts and domestic concerns. The prescribed ritual, which first included personal cleansing, was followed by the performance of an animal sacrifice. The patient would then lie down in the appropriate part of the sanctuary, either in the *abaton* or, in the case of the Amphiareion at Oropus, the *stoa*. The god would appear to the patient in a dream and would give specific advice. For a graphic presentation of such a dream, see the stele of Archinos of Oropus,

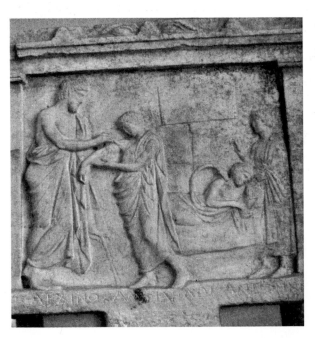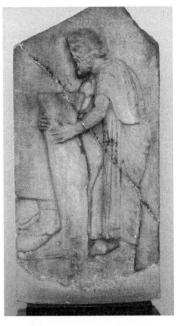

10 Left a) A fourth-century BC votive relief depicting the god Amphiaraus curing a young man, Archinus of Oropus; *right* b) A votive relief is offered to a deity of healing. *From the National Archaeological Museum, Athens*

(*10a*). Here the incubation as it was practised in the domain of the healing gods is depicted. The relief is dated to the fourth century BC. It represents the healing of the injured shoulder of a young man, Archinos of Oropus, by the god, through the lick of a snake during a dream. Two or three scenes from the episode are shown at once and it is difficult to interpret their proper sequence and meaning with certainty. However, the god's resemblance to the iconography of Asclepius is quite striking, possibly representing the 'type' of a healer rather than a portrait. The following lines (649-732) from Aristophanes' play *Wealth*, or *Plutus*, are informative:

> Anyway, the temple servant put out all the lamps and told us to go to sleep, warning us to remain silent if we heard any noise. So we all lay there quietly; but I could not sleep. There was an old woman with a pot of wheat broth lying near her head, and I was struck by this and I had a consuming desire to creep up on that pot. So I looked up, and what did I see but a priest taking the cheese-cakes and figs off the holy table; after which he went all round the altars seeing if anyone had left a cake there, and he consecrated all of them by putting them into his bag. Well, that assured me that what I intended to do was an act of the highest piety, so I got up and made for the pot of broth.

As described by Aristophanes, the offerings placed on the god's altar consisted of such simple things as cakes, bakemeats and figs. When the god appeared, ceremonies were performed. Asclepius would prescribe the therapy, whether herbal medicine, exercise or hot and cold baths. He would also name the sacrifice required. This was rarely onerous or expensive but at each sanctuary the sacrifice was different. In Cyrene goats were offered[19] but at Epidaurus these were banned.[20] Oxen and stuffed pigs are recorded.[21] Cockerels were also allowed: note the last words of Socrates after swallowing the hemlock – 'send a cock to Asclepius'.[22] When the patient was healed, he was expected to offer the promised sacrifice in thanksgiving and to fulfil any other vows he had made. This may well have been to present a model of the affected part. In Greece examples of such limbs may be seen in the museum at Corinth. Asclepius was known from testimonies carved in stone at his sanctuaries, for his ability to cure all diseases. Physicians were also present at the temples.

THE AMPHIAREION OF OROPUS

A further healing sanctuary of interest with roots in Greek myth and a long history of pilgrimage and use by the sick and disabled is found at Oropus, situated in a pleasant wooded valley thirty miles from Athens (*11* and *12*). During the fifth and fourth centuries BC the Amphiareion at Oropus would have been a site to equal in popularity the sanctuary of Asclepius at Epidaurus. Pausanias relates the story from Greek myth of the seer and divine healer, Amphiaraus.[23] He was a Greek hero of the generation earlier than the Trojan wars, who took part in the expedition of the Seven against Thebes. In the legend, as Amphiaraus was fleeing from a predicted certain death, Zeus cast out a thunderbolt, opening a cleft in the earth in which the hero sheltered with his chariot. As a result of this divine favour, Amphiaraus (the name means twice-holy), became a chthonic deity and functioned in two capacities, as both a divine healer and a prophet. The god performed miraculous cures over several centuries. The sanctuary at Oropus was founded in the last quarter of the fifth century BC and was at once an oracular shrine and a health spa. Under Roman state patronage, it attained added importance, particularly in the first century BC when the games flourished, encouraged by money supplied by Sulla.[24] The statue bases of Brutus and an equestrian portrait statue of Marcus Agrippa provide evidence for the continuation of the site into the very end of the Republic and beyond.

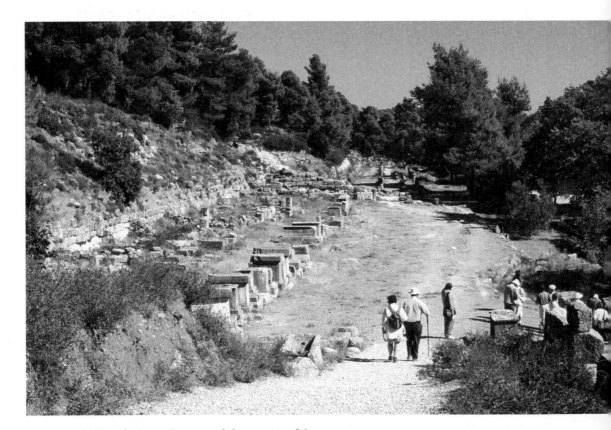

11 Temple site at Oropus and the remains of the stoa

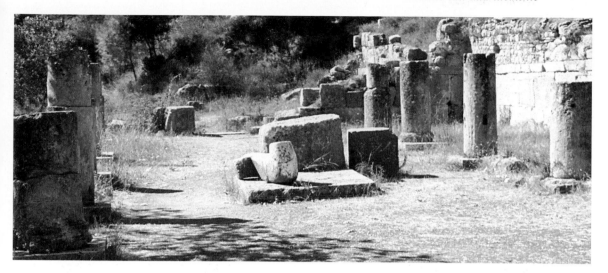

12 The remains of the cult statue at Oropus

THE ARCHAEOLOGY

The sanctuary was first excavated by the Greek archaeological service between 1884 and 1929. After a period of inactivity, sporadic restorations were resumed in 1960.[25] Amphiaraus is believed to have emerged from the underworld through the sacred spring. In ancient times it was forbidden to use this for such mundane, or impure, purposes as personal washing. However, the water was thought to possess medicinal properties which pilgrims were permitted to drink. According to Pausanias, when a person was cured of a disease, or was in receipt an oracular pronouncement, they would drop gold and silver coins into the spring in thanks. Lower down the valley, the water fed into a stream where it could be freely used. Today the remains of the colossal cult statue still lie among the ruins of the temple in which it once stood (*12*).

A large part of the fourth-century theatre, which could accommodate some 3,000 spectators, is also preserved. Five marble thrones with scroll ornaments are present, as well as the proscenium arch. Contests were held in poetry and music and plays. It is known from inscriptions that people wishing to consult the god followed a ritual. First personal purification was necessary and then a ram was sacrificed. Afterwards the patient slept on the fresh skin of the animal to receive either the god's oracular advice, or a direct cure.

The difference between Asclepius, the god of medicine, and Amphiaraus lies in the origins of their therapeutic techniques. Asclepius was taught the art of herbal medicine by the centaur Cheiron through the medicinal plants that grew on Mount Pelion, symbolising the curative powers of nature which he practised. Dream interpretation was undertaken by priests at the sanctuaries

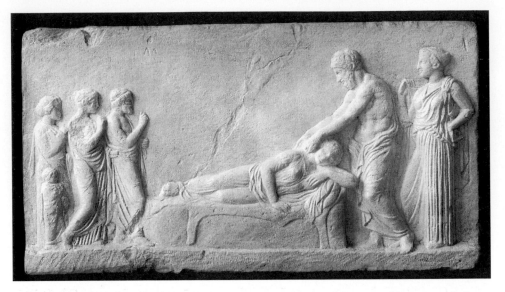

13 Asclepius healing a young girl. The stele demonstrates dream therapy. Marble votive relief, from the Piraeus Asklepieion, early fourth century BC

of Asclepius (*13*) but this was not the same as the dream therapy practised at Oropus. Here the patient was expected to undergo a 'heightened' experience. As a seer and a prophet, the god interpreted dreams but he also gave oracular pronouncements concerning matters other than health, in such subjects as military or athletic events.

Asclepius was different from other gods in the Greek pantheon. He was hardly ever depicted in company with them. Unlike his father, Apollo, his nature was not dualistic; he was benign and kindly and his concern was only with healing. Annual festivals were held in his honour. These were not only serious religious events, they were also occasions of great fun, attended by enormous crowds of people who would participate in games and in theatrical productions, as well as in religious ceremonies and processions. A further attraction would have been the stalls where birds and animals, souvenirs and other items could be bought and sold. According to the Roman writer, Celsus (*De Medicina*, Prooenium 2), 'Asclepius is celebrated as the most ancient authority, and because he cultivated this science (medicine), as yet rude and vulgar, with little more than common refinement, he was numbered among the gods'. The cult of Asclepius continued for more than a thousand years, to be ousted, eventually, by Christianity.

~ 2 ~

GREEK SCIENCE AND MEDICINE

The origins of European thought can be traced to the intellectual movement which began in the Ionian Greek city of Miletus in the sixth century BC. Situated on the west coast of Asia Minor, Miletus was possessed of a wide range of personal and trading contacts with other lands and cultures and, as a result, many of the people were prosperous and self-confident.

Initially three Milesian philosophers are important. First, Thales (*fl. c.*600 BC), who astonished the Greek world by predicting an eclipse of the sun in the year 584 and who, after visiting Egypt, originated the art of geometry. Next, Anaximander (*fl. c.*610-545 BC), the author of the earliest known prose work on nature, in which he attempted to explain the origins of the world and of humankind, perhaps in an attempt to substitute science for myth'.[1] Anaximenes (*fl. c.*546 BC) postulated that air, as opposed to water (contrary to the theory of Thales), was the ultimate constituent of the universe. Furthermore, he saw the universe as disc-like, supported on a cushion of air. Hecataeus (*c.*500 BC), a prominent statesman and geographer, later wrote a work entitled *Genealogies*, perhaps another critical attempt to rationalise the Greek myths.

However, most important is the historian Herodotus (*c.*490-*c.*425 BC). In his great work, *The Histories*, he demonstrates the influence of Homeric oral tradition, in that his sources were mainly verbal and his work was based on witness, on what he could see and what he had heard. Herodotus had a keen eye and ear for marvels and strange customs. Although he was, deservedly, known as the 'Father of History', detractors have called him the 'Father of Lies'. Later accounts from travellers in the sixteenth century, telling their own stories of the wonders of distant places, have partially dispelled that negative view.

33

THE PRE–SOCRATIC PHILOSOPHERS

Coinciding with the rise of democracy, the formation of the city-states and the expansion of the *polis*, the new intellectual movement converged upon Athens. The arrival of philosophers from widely different backgrounds and areas of interest inevitably brought about a priod of great enligthen-ment. Theories originated concerning science, philosophy and medicine, which quickly became separate fields of inquiry and study. The 'atomists', Leucippus (*fl. c.*435 BC) and Democritus (*fl. c.*460 BC) from Abdera, on the Thracian coast, claimed that the essence of the universe was a flux of atoms in a void, an idea which was later embraced by Epicurus (341-271 BC) from Samos. A further interest of Epicurus was in the elimination of superstition. Heraclitus (*fl. c.*491 BC) and his followers came to Greece from Ephesus, bringing ideas of balanced change in a world composed of the elements of fire, air, earth and water. Empedocles (*fl. c.*492-432 BC) from Sicily had a similar but connected idea; he also regarded nature as composed basically of fire, earth, air and water, but for him, these elements were held in a combi-nation of temporary stability.

Empedocles, known as both a scientist and a healer, seems to have been the first to suggest some of the key physiological doctrines in Greek medicine. These included the concept of innate heat as active in the digestive processes. In this system food was thought to become 'cooked' in the stomach. Empedocles also realised the cooling function of breath and supported the notion that blood is manufactured in the liver. Parmenides (*fl. c.*515-after 450 BC), founder of the Eliatic school of philosophy, whose teachings survive in verse, eschewed monocausal theories. He maintained that processes of change and stability were the key questions to be answered. Both Empedocles and Parmenides were supported in their conclusions by Zeno of Elea (*fl. c.*490-after 445 BC), who took over the Eliatic school when the founder moved to Athens, and by Mellisus of Samos. Intellectual discourse was integral to Greek life, and philosophical speculations about nature became merged with medical dialogue concerning health and disease.

The application of philosophical theory to medicine was in large part due to the work of Alcmaeon of Croton (*fl. c.*470 BC). He was the first to believe that the brain and not the heart was the source of human intelligence. This idea was followed by Plato, but not by Aristotle. The brain's function, as it later came to be understood, is described in the Hippocratic treatise, 'On the Sacred Disease', discussed below. Alcmaeon was also the first to set down the doctrine of health as a balance of bodily fluids, later to be called 'the four humours' by the Hippocratics. The theory of humours developed further in the Roman period when it became associated with the four elements, earth, air, fire and water. Moreover, the humoral theory was the basis of classical medicine and it survived at least until the seventeenth century AD. Although few details of the life of Alcmaeon are known, several medical theories are attributed to him, confirming his reputation as an original and independent thinker.

Alcmaeon possessed the same rational outlook as the natural philosophers who preceded him and the Hippocratic philosophers who came after him. His most important discovery occurred when, for some reason, perhaps by means of incision, he performed a direct examination of the eye. Foreshadowing the work of Herophilus and Erasistratus, he found the optic nerve. Subsequently, from further investigations of the nasal and aural passages, he deduced that these, likewise, must be supplied with nerves. Alcmaeon also believed, in common with the early Egyptians, in the theory of pneuma, that 'those *metu* (vessels) which appear to be arteries', contain air. The concept appears in both the Ebers and the Berlin papyri and was an opinion that was held by the Greeks until it was disproved by Galen in the second century AD.

Sophists were attracted to Athens at this time. One of the first to arrive was Anaxagoras (*fl. c.*500-428 BC), mentor to Pericles (*c.*494-429 BC), the Athenian statesman and politician. Sophists were itinerant teachers who travelled about from one city to another giving lectures and instruction for a fee. They taught a wide range of subjects but were best known for their ability to argue a case from either point of view.[2] This group of scholars would meet and discuss the new natural sciences with other resident or itinerant philosophers and healers. They were instrumental in helping to change the character of medicine from a craft, or *technê*, to a more analytical science.

GREEK MEDICINE

Although in the beginning Greek medicine belonged to the category of craft, or *technê*, it later developed in different directions towards the establishment of complementary groups who can be called 'healers' and 'thinkers'.[3] Nutton argues for a plurality of Greek medicines, which makes use of exorcists, religious healers, herb-gatherers and root-cutters, and folk healers, in conjunction with the newly emerging Hippocratics. All these groups were probably co-existing in competition. Another view[4] is of a single medical tradition of speculation and argument in the fifth century. Temkin suggests that some of these new thinkers may have been leech-gatherers, or practitioners of other crafts, who realised the limitations of the practice of medicine without the application of a theory. Connections between the groups would probably have existed in urban areas, but in rural areas where the populations would have been smaller and more isolated, new thinking and attitudes would have arrived slowly, if at all.

History is written by the victors. It is also written by the educated, upper stratum of society. Therefore, it is not known whether the silent majority living in Athens, for example, would have been aware of recent movements in philosophy and medicine. Possibly talk of the new ideas could have been heard in the market-place, or *agora*. The Athenian *agora* was the public square, just off which, the council, or *boule*, met. It was both a forum for debate and the centre for government, law and commerce. There, in the words of the comic poet Eubulus – a poet of Old Greek comedy, and a contemporary of Aristophanes – people could have found:[5]

> …everything sold together in the same place in Athens: figs, witnesses to summonses, bunches of grapes, turnips, pears, apples, givers of evidence, roses, medlars, porridge, honeycombs, horse-chestnuts, chick peas, law suits, bee-stings puddings, myrtle, allotment machines, irises, lambs, water clocks, laws and indictments.
>
> Eubulus, fr.74

Although the humour is directed against the law, the poet draws a fine picture of the variety of life in the *agora*. Philosophers, healers and sophists may also have proclaimed their wares in that place and, perhaps, the latest medical treatises, herbal cures, or sticks of ointment were available too.

PHYSICIANS, HEALERS AND SCHOOLS OF MEDICINE

In the late sixth century BC, when Asclepius was already known as the god of medicine, but before the advent of Hippocrates (*c*.460–370 BC), two Greek city-states were famous for their doctors and their medical 'schools'. However, such schools bear no resemblance to modern medical schools. They were simply groups of thinkers of similar intellectual persuasions, who gathered together to teach and discuss. The different groups would have possessed their own individual doctrines and theories. Herodotus (3.131-4) tells us that the best doctors were found at Croton in southern Italy, where an early temple of Asclepius was also known, and the next best school was at Cyrene (4.150-8) in modern Libya. The Greek school of medicine at Cnidus on the mainland of Asia Minor, which flourished before the foundation of the Hippocratic school at Cos, taught a similar concept of disease to that held by the Egyptians. In the early fifth century, Cos, celebrated as the birthplace of Hippocrates, also possessed a medical school.

Generally, Greek doctors practised privately, although some were employed by the city-state. The employment of public doctors, *archiatroi*, is known at this early date, although little can be discovered concerning the conditions of their work. Some were permanently resident in their own city, whilst others were itinerant. No institution yet existed whereby a doctor was required to be licensed, nor was special training required. A person in any of the different groups practising healing could practise medicine for a fee and, furthermore, there were no 'official' professional governing bodies to whom they were answerable for mistakes or misconduct. However, the Hippocratic Oath gives an insight into what doctors may, or may not, have been able to take upon themselves to do. It is also possible to infer from it the pitfalls of unprofessional behaviour to which a doctor might be susceptible. Little is known about the origins of the Oath; however, it is known that it was not required to be sworn by all doctors.

the oath provides moral instruction

THE OATH

religious

I swear by Apollo the healer, by Asclepius, by Hygea and all the powers of healing, and call to witness all the gods and goddesses that I may keep this Oath and Promise to the best of my ability and judgement.

I will pay the same respect to my master in the Science as to my parents and share my life with him and pay all my debts to him. I will regard his sons as my brothers and teach them the Science, if they desire to learn it, without fee or contract. I will hand on precepts, lectures and all other learning to my sons, to those of my master, and to those pupils duly apprenticed and sworn, and to none other.

idea of knowledge passed through father - son

I will use my power to help the sick to the best of my ability and judgement; I will abstain from harming or wronging any man by it.

I will not give a fatal draught to anyone if I am asked, nor will I suggest any such thing. Neither will I give a woman means to procure an abortion.

I will be chaste and religious in my life and in my practice.

I will not cut, even for the stone, but I will leave such procedures to the practioners of that craft.

dissection is scorned/prohibited / operation

Whenever I go into a house, I will go to help the sick and never with the intention of doing harm or injury. I will not abuse my position to indulge in sexual contacts with the bodies of women or of men, whether they be freemen or slaves.

Whatever I see or hear, professionally or privately, which ought not to be divulged, I will keep secret and tell no one.

confidentiality

If, therefore, I observe this Oath and do not violate it, may I prosper both in my life and in my profession, earning good repute among all men for all time. If I transgress and forswear this Oath, may my lot be otherwise.

- instructive
- authoritive
- stood test of time

THE ATHENIAN PLAGUE

It may be possible to find influences of contemporary medical theory in a document the overt purpose of which was moral and historical, namely Thucydides' description of the plague of Athens in his *History of the Peloponnesian War* (2.47-55).[6] It is a curious fact, however, that other writers in the Greek world who could have refered to it did not do so. Thucydides' stated purpose was to describe the disease fully enough so that, if it should ever return, it would be recognised. As a result of the scientific detail contained in

instructive/informative

the account, what amounts almost to an 'industry' of modern scholarly papers dealing with the event has arisen. These mainly focus on questions of diagnoses using modern categories of disease. The name of the plague itself remains unrecognised, although DNA studies of ancient skeletal material continue. However, this is not the aspect of Thucydides' chronicle that is of concern here.

In 430 BC, when Athenian culture and power were at their height, the city of Athens was at war with Sparta and its allies. The Peloponnesian wars lasted from 431-404 BC. Within the city walls, on the instructions of Pericles, more than 20,000 people, residents and refugees, were crowded together for protection, while their enemies attacked the countryside. They lived in squalid conditions, in small huts and tents. More refugees were pouring in through the port of Piraeus. Thucydides suspected that the plague had been carried to Athens from Egypt, Libya and the Persian Empire. It first erupted in Athens in the early summer of 430 BC with great loss of life. Subsiding in 429, it broke out again in 427. The crowded, insanitary conditions within the city walls had been ideally suited to the incubation of whatever was the causal organism. Although Thucydides could not identify the plague, his vivid account of the symptoms and progress of the disease is detailed and harrowing.

In keeping with Hippocratic tradition, Thucydides described what he saw, concentrating on prognosis rather than diagnosis. He was interested in explanations for the causes of the plague, such as bad air or even the possibility of poisoned water. The death-rate was high; about a third of the population was lost. The Peace of Nicias was concluded in 421 and, when this failed, people, including Thucydides, blamed the gods, perhaps recalling the plague-scene at the opening of the *Iliad*.

Pericles died in the plague and Athens lost the long war with Sparta, the Periclean Golden Age came to an end. Athenians searched for more effective gods and in 420 BC Asclepius was invited to come to Athens. The god arrived some ten years after the great pestilence had passed. There had been no official action to bring him to Athens as there was to be later in plague-ridden Rome, perhaps a reflection of different political systems. Official recognition of Asclepius at Athens, according to inscriptions, did not occur until 350 BC. It is, however, possible that there was an earlier introduction, perhaps a private healing, in connection with the poet and dramatist Sophocles.

Thucydides' chronicle of the symptoms and effects of the disease may have been exaggeration, or a patriotic justification for political events, but he provides much more than this. He presents, some would argue, the very first realisation of the phenomenon of contagion, although the mechanism was not understood. Thucydides himself was afflicted by the plague and recovered. He noted that those who responded to the ties of friendship and had the courage to visit the sick, likewise tended to suffer from the disease. He recorded that at the siege of Potidaea the soldiers there caught the disease from Hagnon's forces – the plague was carried by people. He describes acquired immunity '…for no one had the disease twice…'. There were, however, those who suffered a second, 'not fatal' form of the disease. As for the effect on society, 'the plague caused a state of unprecedented lawlessness,' and the overall effect was chaos.

In Athens, and later in Rome, educated men were expected to know about medicine. The literature available to them would, conjecturally, have contained a significant medical component. In sum, as described above, the latest treatise from the medical 'schools' may have been in circulation; public debates and medical pamphlets could also have been at hand in the market-place. Thucydides' account demonstrates knowledge of medicine as well as an awareness of Hippocratic humoral theory: 'the year was free from all other kinds of illnesses'. This is a reminder of the Hippocratic treatise 'Epidemics'.[7] His appreciation of the importance of patterns of symptoms is also apparent. Thucydides' contribution to medicine lies in his acute observation of the process of acquired immunity. In addition, his recording of these rationalist ideas demonstrates their availability and use at an early stage in medical history.[8]

HIPPOCRATES

In the first century AD, the Roman writer Celsus was to record in his *De Medicina*:

> It was… Hippocrates of Cos, a man first and foremost worthy to be remembered, notable both for professional skill and for eloquence, who separated this branch of learning from the study of philosophy'.
>
> *Prooemium*, 6-8

As a result of influences from philosophy, the character of Greek medicine changed, becoming more rational, between the fifth and third centuries. The collection of treatises known as the *Hippocratic Corpus* was a result of this movement. Hippocrates was a physician, who eventually became known as the 'Father of Medicine'. He lived a long life during the fifth to the fourth centuries on the island of Cos. The treatises attributed to him were written by a number of different authors. The *Hippocratic Corpus* comprised more than sixty treatises gathered together over a period, whose chronology extends for more than one life-time.

THE HIPPOCRATIC CORPUS

Almost all of the texts are thought to have been compiled between *c.*430 and *c.*330 BC, although some could be later. It seems that around 250 BC they were

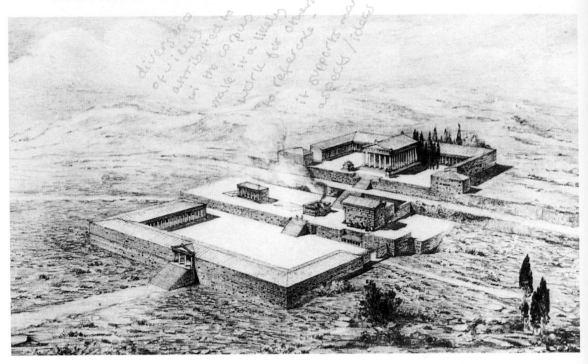

14 The Asklepieion at Cos. *R. Herzog, 1932*

assembled by a librarian in Alexandria and labelled 'Hippocrates'. Although no generalisation can be used to cover all the texts in the *Corpus*, the main thesis which runs through many of them is that in order to know the whole it is first necessary to understand the parts. This is also implicit in the classic Greek injunction to first 'know thyself', referred to earlier. The *Corpus* constituted the basis for the development of western medical ethics from ancient times until the nineteenth century. Some of the treatises held widely divergent views, perhaps suggesting rivalry between the different schools. Hippocrates' own school was at Cos (*14, colour plate 7*).

Hippocratics did not ask 'who' caused diseases, as in the old days when blame was placed firmly in the laps of the gods. Instead, they attempted to define the cause and process of disease by the application of a theory. The humoral theory is the key to Hippocratic medicine. In the earliest stages of its formulation, the body was thought to consist of fluids, or humours. These were blood, phlegm, yellow bile and black bile. The 'humours' determined constitution, temperament and health, whilst the 'pneuma', or air, was the source of consciousness and thought, perception and sensation. Health required harmony and balance between the humours. The condition of the body could also vary between wet/dry, hot/cold, sweet/bitter, and so on. Disease was regarded as a disturbance in the balance of fluids. A humour which became separated in this way was regarded as potent and harmful, since its power was no longer checked by its being compounded with other humours or powers. For example, winter colds were attributed to too much phlegm, and the cause of summer dysentery and vomiting was an excess of bile.

Belonging to the theory of pneuma was the idea that illnesses were attributable to gases. It was thought that disease was due to putrefying residues of food carried in the bowels making gases which permeated and poisoned the body. This idea also largely informed Egyptian medicine, where, as Herodotus (2.79) informs us, purgation was a way of life. The theory led to the continual use of purges by the Greeks in order to rid the body of 'residues' (called 'superfluities' by the school at Cnidus). Indeed, many of the Hippocratic treatments relied on physical intervention in various forms, including the use of evacuative medicines such as hellebore for purgation. Although Hippocratics forbade cutting 'even for bladder stone', other doctors performed such surgery and much else besides, including surgical operations for cataract. Incision of the veins for blood-letting was a much-used practice of humoral therapy (*15*). Hippocratics were also interested in the environment, in ethnography and in far away places and peoples, as well as in epidemics and plagues. Hence, in the treatise 'Airs, Waters, Places' the author attributes differing national characteristics and personality traits to the effects of the elements upon the humours.

Hippocratics were quick to criticise the irrational, expressing scorn for earlier practices which were based on blame, superstition and the necessity for placating the gods. This is best demonstrated in the treatise 'On the Sacred Disease' where the author firmly repudiates 'witch doctors, faith healers, quacks and charlatans'. In this tract, epilepsy is attributed to natural causes, such as an excessive secretion of phlegm in the brain. The idea that epileptic fits occur as a form of divine punishment, or that the disease itself was the direct will of the gods, or the fault of the stars, is dismissed as absurd. Epilepsy, asserted the Hippocratics, was no more difficult to understand, and

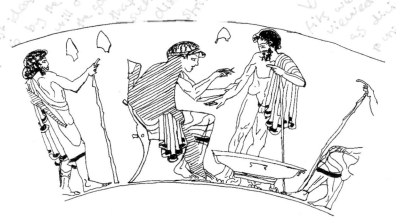

15 Incision of veins for blood-letting in humoral therapy. Cupping vessels hang on the wall. Vase painting, *c.*470 BC

no more or less sacred than any other disease. In chapter 11 the humoral theory is combined with the environmental theory; 'infants who suffer from this disease usually die if the phlegm is copious and the weather is southerly'. The following excerpt is taken from chapter 17 of the treatise:

> It ought to be generally known that the source of our pleasure, merriment, laughter and amusement, as of our grief, pain, anxiety and tears, is none other than the brain. It is especially the organ which enables us to think, see and hear, and to distinguish the ugly and the beautiful, the bad and the good, pleasant and unpleasant. Sometimes we judge according to convention; at other times according to the perceptions of expediency. It is the brain too, which is the seat of madness and delirium, of fears and frights which assail us, often in the night, but sometimes even in the day; it is there where lies the cause of insomnia and sleepwalking, of thoughts that will not come, forgotten duties and eccentricities. All such things result from an unhealthy condition of the brain; it may be warmer than it should be, or it may be colder, or moister or drier, or in any other abnormal state. Moistness is the cause of madness for when the brain is abnormally moist it is necessarily agitated and this agitation prevents sight and hearing being steady. Because of this, varying visual and acoustic sensations are produced, while the tongue can only describe things as they appear and sound. So long as the brain is still, a man is in his right mind... I therefore assert that the brain is the interpreter of comprehension.[9]

The treatise *'On Regimen'* covers what is known in modern times as 'preventative' medicine: 'In the first place,... if sick men fared just as well eating and drinking and living exactly as healthy men do... there would be little need for the science of medicine'.[10] The treatise *'Tradition in Medicine'* is an explanation of the empirical basis of medicine, written in the fifth century BC. The physician was supposed to maintain health by tailoring the patient's diet, exercise and rest. *Regimen* also dictated the way the person should sleep, dream and react to the environment. Eating too much or too little food, or taking in too much or too little fluid, particularly wine, disturbed the balance of the humours. Correct or incorrect diet determined health and disease; these were within the will of the individual. There was, therefore, a moral dimension to the practice of *regimen*: 'A man ought to realise that health is his most valued possession and learn how to treat his illness by his own judgement'.[11]

EGYPTIAN MEDICINE

Egypt, both in its society and its organisations, is different from Greek and Roman cities and provinces. Therefore, in order to properly introduce Egyptian medicine, a short history is required.

Medicine developed early in Egypt, due, perhaps, to its unique environment and topography. It was a closed system, the country itself being an isolated oasis situated between two formidable desert areas. The Nile Valley, a cleft between the two areas, was easily defended, giving rise to long-term stability and independence. The River Nile provided the Ancient Egyptians with their theory of the body and of disease. Its annual inundation caused unlimited supplies of water bearing rich silts to gush over the land. Farmlands received the water through irrigation channels which sometimes became blocked. Therefore, by careful observation of nature, the Egyptians found ways to care for themselves. They drew the parallel that, like the channels of the Nile, the human system could also become blocked by putrefying substances (*wekhedu*); these were transported by the *metu*, or vessels, and were the cause of disease. This idea formed the basis of Ancient Egyptian medical thought.

Several types of primary sources exist for the study of medical practice in Ancient Egypt. These include evidence from papyri, tomb bas-reliefs, human remains and the writings of Greek historians, notably Herodotus. The sources tell of an educated society interested in things scientific and medical. Medicine in Egypt was already an ancient craft when the Homeric poems were composed, as seen in the *Odyssey* (IV.226-32).

In the Ptolemaic period, Imhotep became identified by the Greeks and Romans with Asclepius (*16*). A shrine was built for him at the temple of Hatshepsut in Deir el-Bahri which quickly became a place of pilgrimage. Although Imhotep was addressed in an inscription on a private statue as 'one who comes to the one who calls to him to cast off sickness and heal the body', his tomb has not, so far, been found and it is not known for certain that he was a physician, a *swnw*.[12]

Of all the discoveries made by archaeologists over many seasons of excavations in Egypt, among the most important are the medical papyri. At least twelve of these were discovered during the nineteenth and early twentieth centuries. Glosses found on the texts made by early scholars have been useful to modern translators. The Ebers papyrus and the Edwin Smith papyrus (*17*) are dated to approximately the same period, *c.*seventeenth-sixteenth centuries BC. The principal document, the Ebers papyrus, is from Thebes. It is astonishing to note that, although the Greeks are normally credited with being the first to make recorded medical case-histories, at this early period in Egyptian history, insights are provided into individual illnesses and ancient pharmacy. Over 800 remedies, including plant extracts, animal organs, minerals and magic are described, ranging from drastic treatments for the removal of putrefying residues in the gut and bowel, to chants and the use of amulets.

The Ebers papyrus contains a long section on diagnosis and treatment. This included preparations for treating crocodile bites and boils; goats' dung mixed with fermenting yeast could be spread on a poultice for treating burns, and scribes' excrement, mixed with fresh milk was applied to boils. Such ingredients would have been highly regarded for their apotropaic value. Treatments recommended for localised inflammatory conditions consisted of crushed onion with honey taken in beer, or a chopped bat on a poultice.[13] Ancient peoples believed that diseases which were common in damp places and would respond to the plants which thrived in such places; willow was such a plant. In any case the treatment would have been effective since willow contains salicylic acid, the basis of aspirin, a drug which quickly alleviates pain and inflammation.[14] A description of the treatment of an infected wound with leaves or root of willow appears below:

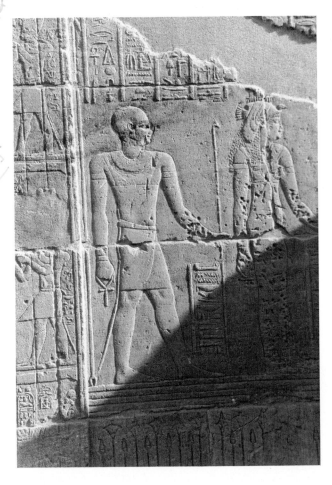

16 Imhotep at the temple of Philae

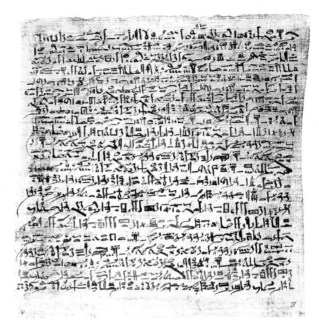

17 The Edwin Smith Surgical Papyrus. The photograph is of the fifth column of the papyrus. Vol. 1, the transcription and commentary, shows that this includes: case 9 (pp. 217-24), referring to a wound in the forehead producing a comminuted fracture of the skull; case 10 (pp. 225-33), referring to a gaping wound at the top of the eyebrow, which penetrates to the bone; case 11 (pp. 234-44), referring to a broken nose; case 12 (pp. 244-51), referring to a break in the nasal bone and to the setting of the bone

> When you examine a man with an irregular wound... and that wound is inflamed... [there is] a concentration of heat; the lips of that wound are reddened and that man is hot in consequence... Then you must make cooling substances for him to draw the heat out... leaves of the willow.

The Ebers papyrus is also the main source for information concerning treatment for eye diseases in ancient Egypt. The eye was an important symbol in Egyptian mythology. For instance, the eye of Horus torn out by Seth was magically restored by Thoth. The magical, restored eye then became a powerful apotropaic amulet and is often worn as such today.[15]

> To drive away inflammation of the eyes, grind the stems of the juniper of Biblos, steep them in water, apply to the eyes of the sick person and he will be quickly cured. To cure granulations of the eye prepare a remedy of collyrium, verdigris, onions, blue vitriol, powdered wood; mix and apply to the eyes.

Incantations were recommended for watering of the eye; this could have been due to a number of causes. In the condition of trachoma the eylashes turn inwards, scratching and causing injury to the coverings of the eye, with an infectious watery discharge of pus. It was endemic in Egypt, as in other parts of the ancient world. Today the condition persists in parts of Africa and Asia where poor living conditions mean that the eyes become permanently infected and blindness is a frequent result (*18*). Besides reference to ingrown lashes, cataracts and burst blood vessels are also described. Only a few of the therapies recommended in the papyrus would have been beneficial, or even soothing. In the Roman period more effective prescriptions (in addition to surgical instruments (*19*)) were available.

The Edwin Smith papyrus, second in length to the Ebers, appears to be a surgical treatise. Its form is that of a systematic progression through the body from head to toe, *de capite ad calcem*, and from front to back. Unlike the Ebers papyrus, it is almost devoid of magic. Its original purpose is unclear; perhaps it was a standard reference for the treatment of trauma, or possibly a teaching aid. Not only is there a classic account of dislocation of the jaw together with the method used for reducing this, there is also treatment for the reduction of a dislocated shoulder. Moreover, skeletal examples of well-healed fractures with good alignment of parts are sometimes discovered in archaeological contexts, such as those in Nubia, where palm splints were found.[16]

In the seventh-sixth centuries BC the land of Egypt was at peace and commerce flourished. At last the xenophobic Egyptians allowed Greek traders and mercenaries to establish an *emporion* on the Nile Delta; it was called Naucratis. Herodotus (2.178-9) is the primary source for the history of the site. By this time, the period of intense speculation concerning natural science and philosophy had begun in the Greek world and exchanges of ideas and technology, with inevitable, if uneasy, intermixing of the two cultures, would have occurred. For example Greeks are known to have patronised Egyptian gods of healing. A short time before the establishment of the Hippocratic 'school' in Cos, teachers of the 'school' at Cnidus (formed in the fifth century BC), emulated the Egyptian habit of purgation and fasting. The practice was based on the idea, originating in Egypt, that disease arises in the bowel. It is possible that some Egyptian medical practices were taken over by the Greeks for they greatly admired Egyptian culture.

Herodotus tells us that Egyptian physicians, unlike Greek doctors, were not known for gentleness (2.80 and 3.134-7). King Darius (*c.*521-486 BC) employed Egyptian physicians in the Persian Court but it was a captive Greek doctor, Democedes, who successfully treated the king for a damaged and diseased ankle, '...by using Greek methods, and substituting milder remedies for the rough-and-ready treatment of the Egyptian doctors, he enabled the king to get some sleep, and very soon cured him completely'. Democedes also successfully treated Darius' wife, Atossa, for an infected breast abscess and in return, with her assistance, he eventually won his freedom and returned to Greece. Democedes is the earliest-known practising physician. His father had been a priest of Asclepius at Cnidus before moving on to Croton in southern Italy. From this it is infered that, in addition to possessing a natural aptitude for healing, the son learnt his medical skills at his father's side and could have been much influenced by temple medical practice.

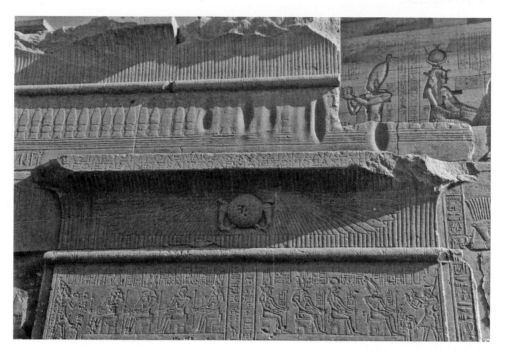

18 Greek inscription of Imhotep. Philae Temple.

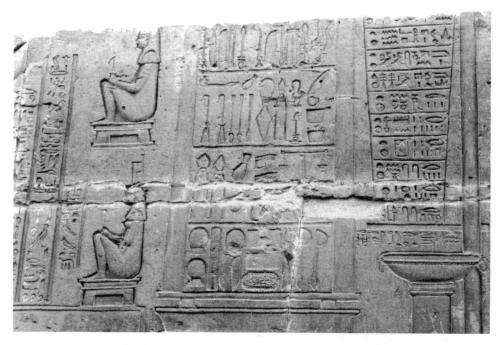

19 The Roman surgical tools at Kom Ombo Temple: these show a variety of recognisable Roman surgical tools and cupping vessels. The women sit on birthing stools

PTOLEMAIC EGYPT

Egypt remained under Persian control until its conquest by the Macedonian king, Alexander the Great, late in 331 BC. Since the age of thirteen, Alexander had been fortunate in having had as tutor the great Aristotle, pupil of Plato. When Alexander died in AD 323, his generals took over different parts of his conquered world. Egypt was governed by Ptolemy, who possessed great personal wealth, which he used to enhance the city of Alexandria.

With the foundation of Alexandria, Greek doctors arrived in Egypt where they could enjoy the benefits of the riches of the country. Many were students of the Hippocratic school at Cos. Alexandria quickly became the major cultural and scientific centre of the Greek and Roman world. The city possessed an immense library, where every book in the known world was copied and kept. This was, of course, largely the result of the Egyptians' monopoly of papyrus. Eventually around 700,000 manuscripts were held in the library, whose amenities also included an observatory, zoological gardens, lecture halls, museum – or hall of the Muses – and rooms for research. The prospect of rich and powerful patronage was a further enticement to scholars from a variety of social and geographical backgrounds. Free thought and experimentation flourished. There was great interest in the natural world, resulting in an increase in knowledge of animals, plants, minerals and drugs. A medical school was established, which achieved a high reputation. In the second century AD, Galen studied anatomy at Alexandria.

Among other physicians who studied and worked in Alexandria were the two great anatomists, Herophilus of Chalcedon (*c.*330–260 BC) and Erasistratus of Ceos (*c.*330–255 BC). Although their texts survive only in fragments, Herophilus wrote at least eleven treatises; they are known from later authors such as Celsus who lived during the reign of the Emperor Tiberius (AD 14–37), and Galen. Herophilus received his medical education from Praxagoras on the island of Cos, whilst Erasistratus studied at Aristotle's Peripatetic school in Athens.

HELLENISTIC MEDICINE

At Alexandria important advances were made, not only in pharmacology, but in the study of anatomy, which, for the first time in history, broke all former barriers and taboos as human dissection was performed on the living and the dead. It is possible that the climate of mummification in Egypt was the catalyst which allowed this to happen. Celsus (*De Med. Prooemium* 23–6) writes: '… they laid open men whilst alive, criminals received out of the prison from the kings, and whilst they were still breathing, observed parts which hitherto nature had concealed…'. Whether or not this is true, it cannot be disputed that the result of the momentum in anatomy was to vastly increase knowledge and understanding in the subject, as internal organs were observed in action and parts were named.

Herophilus conducted investigations into the brain and the nervous system, and into the vascular systems and the pulse; he discovered the prostate gland and the testes and the manufacture therein of the semen. In the female reproductive system Herophilus demonstrated the Fallopian tubes and the ovaries. During his dissections of the eye he discovered and named the four tunics of that small organ. Devoting an entire treatise to the topic, he devised a technical nomenclature for the different parts of the eye, which was based on items of everyday use. For example, the net-like third tunic of the eye is retiform, hence *retina*. The posterior surface of the iris he described as 'like the skin of a grape'. Herophilus discovered that arteries carried blood, not air. In this discovery he modified the work of Praxagolas his great tutor in Cos, who believed the arteries served as channels for *pneuma*, not blood; he established the differences between the blood vessels, and between veins and arteries. He also dissected animals, as shown by his description of the *rete mirabile*, the network of arteries found at the base of the brain in animals, though not present in humans. Erasistratus not only recognised the heart as a pump, he also identified the action of the valves. Indeed, he came very close to Harvey's theory of the circulation of the blood. He regarded the brain as the seat of intelligence, and he distinguished its different parts and described the motor and sensory nerves. Erasistratus was more a physiologist than an anatomist. He rejected the theory that the processes of digestion involved 'cooking' the food in the stomach and postulated the theory of peristalsis.

However, thirty years later, the practice of human dissection in Alexandria stopped as suddenly as it had begun. The reasons for this are unknown. Most probably it was due to the domination of one of the competing sects, the Empirics, which formed during this period. As far as it is known, human dissection was not practised again until the seventeenth century with the advent of Vesalius. Nevertheless, considerable changes had occurred as a result of the new research. In the first place surgery became a specialism in its own right and this led to the development of other specialist fields of study in medicine. A further benefit was the evolution of a scientific language and the formation of the first truly scientific medical teaching centre.

Following the Alexandrian anatomy period, medicine, like philosophy, split into further sects (see p.197). Herophilus and Eristratus consolidated the Dogmatic school which approved dissection and stressed the importance of research and theory. Their opponents, the Empirics, were dismissive of dissection and the search for hidden causes, preferring the physician to work from experience and analogy. Once Greek medicine became established in Rome, a new sect, who called themselves 'Methodists', led by Asclepiades of Bithynia, formed an opposition to the Dogmatists. The Empirics advocated treatment with astringent medicines and laxatives, or *regimen*. Whereas all the sects had found support for their theories in the *Hippocratic Corpus*, the Methodists rejected the complicated humoral theory. A fourth sect developed from a split with the Dogmatists and called themselves the 'Pneumatists'. They reverted to the theories of *pneuma* and the four humours. At the end of the second and first centuries BC these four schools were prominent and active. Indeed, they spanned the main period when Greek medicine encountered Rome (for further elucidation of this aspect of ancient medicine see pp.197-8). At the same time, medical literature became more readily available, with the writings of, among others, Celsus, Pliny, Dioscorides, Rufus of Ephesus (AD 70-120) and Soranus (*fl. c.*AD 100). Areteus of Cappadocia (*fl.* AD 140) and Galen (*c.*AD 129-216?), were followed by other writers. Alongside all this activity a lively temple medicine flourished.

☙ 3 ❧

MATERIA MEDICA,
OR THE MATERIALS OF MEDICINE

When Greece surrendered she took control of her rough invader, and brought the arts to rustic Latium. Then the primitive metre of Saturn dried up and the fetid smell gave way to cleaner air; nevertheless for many years there remained, and still remain today, signs of the farmyard. It was late when the Roman applied his brains to Greek writing. In the peace which followed the Punic wars he began to wonder if Aeschylus, Thespis and Sophocles had anything useful to offer, and if he himself could produce an adequate version. He tried, and liked the result, having grand ideas and a natural keenness. (He did catch some of the tragic spirit and his strokes came off, but he had the novice's guilty dread of using a rubber.)

Horace, *Epistles* 2.1.156-67, tr. N. Rudd

I said that the cure itself is a certain leaf, but in addition to the drug, there is a certain charm, which if someone chants when he makes use of it, the medicine altogether restores him to health, but without the charm there is no profit from the leaf.

Plato, *Charmides*, 155E, trans. R.R. Sprague

In this chapter Rome's conquest of the Hellenistic world, in so far as it concerns medicine, is considered and the quotations with which it opens provide a link between both Greek and Roman cultures. Indeed, the use of charms or incantations was a practice common to peoples in ancient civilisations. In Plato's *Republic* (426b) incantations are included with 'medicaments, cauteries and operations' as possible therapies available to physicians. Although some readers may be tempted to smile at the notion, such effects of the human voice will now be discussed in the light of modern psychological understanding.

The use and potential power of words in charms or incantation (also known as *epode*, *logos kalos* or song, here regarded as interchangeable), have already been seen in Homer, in the *epode* with which the sons of Autolycus heal the wounds of Odysseus, and also in Egyptian medicine for the treatment of infected eyes. Reference to this art, by implication magical, while often therapeutic, is frequently met with in ancient texts; therefore, some discussion of it is required. Although in the Hippocratic treatise 'On the Sacred Disease', incantation is regarded as one of the 'ignorant practices with which witch doctors, quacks and charlatans' surround the diagnosis and treatment of epilepsy, others have written of it differently. In the view of Entralgo,[1] nowhere is incantation better observed than in the works of Plato, who makes many references to the subject.

Throughout his life as a writer, from the early *Charmides* to the *Laws*, Plato held the view that the spoken word was superior to the written word. He explored the power of the chant, or incantation, in both its negative and positive aspects. It is the positive, therapeutic use of the incantation that is of concern here. In the *Theaetetus* (149c), Plato speaks of the midwives' ability to excite or to relieve the pains of childbirth by the recitation of charms or beautiful speeches. Fear of death is discussed in the *Phaedo* (77e) where it is said to be a 'childish' fear, easily dispelled by the daily use of a chant.

Turning to the *Charmides*, Socrates, upon his return from the Battle of Potidaea, meets young Charmides in the gymnasium and agrees to cure him of a headache. Socrates knows of an effective cure; it is a certain plant to which it is necessary to add a charm. Although the dialogue contains much more than this (it is actually a device for introducing a philosophical discussion) one of its main points is that good physicians always treat the disease of the part by ministering with suitable *regimen* to the whole person. The body cannot be treated without treating the soul, or the *psyche* – the mind of the patient. This is treated with charms, beautiful speeches, or incantations.

DO WORDS HAVE POWER?

The *epode* or chant itself consists of a formula of magical character, the content of which varies according to circumstances. It was sung or recited in the presence of the patient in order to bring about a cure. The simplest form was a direct appeal to the disease itself. Sometimes a deity, or deities, were invoked and at others the *epode* was linked to a particular disease and to the use of a prescribed plant remedy. In the *Charmides*, Socrates states that for the plant cure to be effective, the practitioner should first use the chant. This would reinforce the effectiveness of the medicinal plant remedy. Incantations, or song, were especially to be relied upon when treating chronic illness.

For an early Roman view of the power of words, we turn to Cato (234–149 BC). His work 'On Agriculture' was an informative notebook concerning the

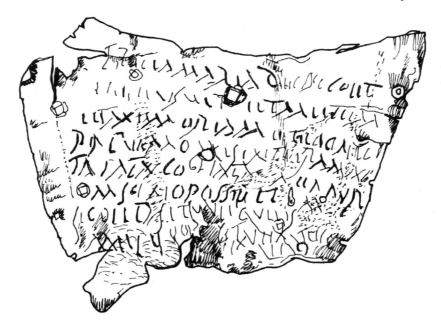

20 A lead Curse Tablet from London shows contemporary attitudes to the human body. It reads, 'I curse Tretia Maria and her life and mind and memory: thus may she be unable to speak what things are concealed, not be able to...' (the reading is by R.G. Collingwood, 1965).

duties of the farmer in the days of the Republic. In it (CLX), Cato claims, 'any kind of dislocation can be cured by a charm'. Besides a specific formula, his charm involves a ceremony with a green reed and a knife. Varro (116-27 BC) likewise, 'On Agriculture', I.ii.25-8, knew of a charm to cure painful feet, perhaps caused by gout, or podagra. This was chanted 'thrice nine' times. In the ancient world (as also today in the Judaeo-Christian scriptures) there is power in the number three, also in the number seven and in multiples of these numbers – as well as in the use of saliva, fasting and nakedness.[2] Varro's cure for painful feet consists of touching the ground and spitting on it, followed by the words, 'Earth take the pest to thee, Health tarry here with me!' The patient would be fasting whilst he chanted and the pain would then go into the ground.

Pliny the Elder (c.AD 23-79) in his *Natural History* (XXVIII.iii) discusses incantations at greater length and possibly more 'scientifically'. For, to the question, 'Have words and formulated incantation power?' he finds: 'as individuals, all our wisest men reject belief in them although, as a body, the public at all times believes in them unconsciously'. Pliny adds to this, 'there is power in ritual formulae...'. He includes prayers to the gods, who, as he says, would expect the recitation of the formulae to be word-perfect. On superstitions in general, Pliny informs us that 'the effect of omens is really in our own control and their influence is conditional on the way we receive each'.

The chant or incantation in itself cannot be dismissed as a purely magical or superstitious practice, nor should its power be underestimated. People have always responded to the sound of the human voice, from the pleasing effect of the Homeric *aoidos*, the singer of epic, to the theatre of ancient Greece, and no less in theatre and song, or threnody, today. This may be placebo in part, but it is also more than that. For, as well as experiencing pleasure, the patient receives other benefits. Similarly, today it is well known that the doctor, nurse or physiotherapist who takes time to talk to patients is more effective than the one who silently reaches for the prescription pad. In the case of children, too, many benefits are gained from reading to them, especially before sleep, when the power of the human voice often dispels a child's fears of the night. Ordinary daily discourse teaches us that words have a power and life of their own, whether they are spoken or written or sung. Words also accumulate a mystical aura, evidenced from antiquity down to the present time both in religious ceremony and in books, especially those for children.

INSCRIBED CHARMS

Following the suggestion that power is intrinsic to the spoken word, attention now turns to the written form of the charm. This may take the shape of an inscribed magical text, possibly, by-passing the need for complex rituals and knowledge of drugs. The ever-present inscribed formula, carried on the person, would make for a more constant relationship between the charm itself and the patient. This relationship may or may not have included the one who inscribed

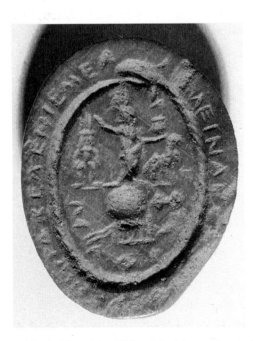
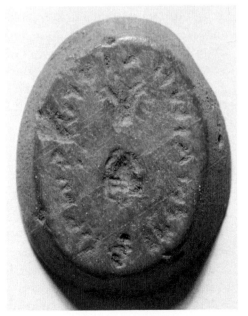

21 Both sides of the Dicket Mead haematite amulet

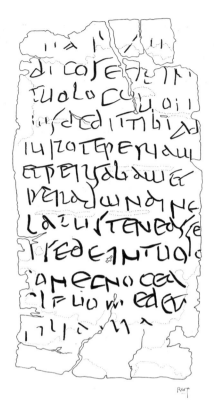

22 The lead tablet
from West Deeping

the charm. The social context would have been different, too, for an inscription speaks of a more literate person than the folk-healer or the root-cutter.[3]

An example of a large class of Graeco-Egyptian inscribed charms can be seen in the small Graeco-Egyptian haematite amulet (*21, colour plate 10*) from the Romano-British site at Dicket Mead, near the Lockley's Roman villa.[4] Written on the obverse of the amulet is an invocation against the daemon Typhon, a powerful elemental force, with a conventional representation of the uterus, including the Fallopian tubes and ligaments, as described by Galen. Parallels to this iconographic device are found on similar amulets. All are engraved on blood-red haematite gemstones. The whole design is framed by a serpent devouring its tail, the Egyptian symbol for eternity. The reverse of the Lockley's example bears the sacred beetle, in Egyptian mythology the symbol of creation. Another uterine symbol is below it. Moreover, and most important for the question, 'do words have power?' these images are surrounded by a text cut in Greek capitals, 'ΟΡΩΡΙΟΥΘ, running three times round the whole design which, translated, reads 'Ororiouth', the spirit who gives protection in women's diseases. The charm is repeated to the power of three.

A similar spell, again from Roman Britain, is to be seen on an inscribed lead tablet from Rectory Farm at West Deeping Roman Villa[5] (*22*). The tablet carries thirteen lines of New Roman cursive writing which reads, 'Womb, I invoke you, stay in your place... has given to you. I adjure you by Iao, and by Saboa and by Adona, not to hold on to the side; but to stay in your place, and not to hurt Cleuomedes daughter of A[...]'. These are names of gods who gave protection in women's ailments. They are of Hebraic origin. In Roman Britain, amulets invoking Iaô are found at Silchester, Great Chesters, and Thetford. Additional interest in the case of the Rectory Farm text is found in the name 'Cleuomedes', which is a Greek name; here, then, is the same Graeco-Egyptian magic, but translated into Latin.[6]

Other medications and therapies were available: religious medicine included pilgrimage to the god at his sanctuary. Alternatively, the patient could choose a visit to a Greek doctor, or a consultation with a herbalist or root-cutter, at a stall or shop in the market-place. A further option was a prognostication, perhaps, sought from an augur. The itinerant healer, making his perambulations, would possibly incorporate a home visit. Such healers were found everywhere in Roman towns and, to a lesser degree, in the countryside too. All were in competition, intent on making a living. In rural areas, people produced their own herbs, but in towns they would obtain supplies from ships trading in drugs, which sailed around the Mediterranean and on the high seas to India or China. Marine archaeology has uncovered wrecks on which supplies of medical equipment were found.[7] These included plants and prepared drugs, in addition to medical implements and surgical instruments. Treatment with various herbs, spices and metals would have been combined with temple medicine. In the so-called medical market place where there was a plurality of health workers people were at liberty to try any or all of these therapies.

SOURCES

In the quotation with which this chapter began, Plato tells us that of equal value to the *epode* are the herbal remedies supplied by nature. There is no shortage of evidence for medicines made from herbs, animals, insects and minerals in the literary texts, both Greek and Roman. Theophrastus (*c*.371–*c*.287 BC, another 'Father', this time of botany) was a useful primary source for many Greeks and Romans and also Scribonius Largus (*fl. c*.AD 1–50), a near-contemporary of Pliny and Dioscorides. In the *Compositiones*, or Prescriptions, his only surviving work, he uses many herbal remedies, although the list of illnesses to be cured is short compared with that of Pliny and Dioscorides. Very little is known of Celsus (*fl. c*.AD 14–37), whose *De Medicina*, 'On Medicine', is the sole survivor of a much larger encyclopaedia. It, too, provides information concerning plant cures and is a clear account of ancient medicine and surgery much drawn from Greek sources.

The *Natural History* of Pliny is a valuable source for the Roman way of healing within the family, as also is the *De Materia Medica* of Dioscorides (*c.* AD 40-90). Among others, a later writer, Soranus of Ephesus, *c.*AD 100, is discussed below and also Galen; both were major influences on medicine down to modern times. Besides the works of these writers, papyri also provide primary evidence of physicians and medication. This applies in particular to the 'Michigan Medical Codex', which is relevant to the late Roman period. Archaeological evidence for the actual use of plants in medicine is more problematic. Botanical remains, which may indicate medicinal use, are found in courtyards of military hospitals, in watery deposits, in burials and beneath the fallout from volcanoes.

Roman families possessed their own ideas and handed down recipes for ailments. This was a source of great pride when, during the last centuries of the Republic, the confrontation with Greek medicine began. On the Roman farm, *latifundium*, for example, the head of the household, *paterfamilias*, was also the resident physician, with responsibility for the health of all the souls in his home and on his estate. In his own domain this would have been a powerful position which he may have been reluctant to change. According to his means, he would have gathered appropriate knowledge and equipment for use in his household, or in the slave infirmary. He may even have aquired a few surgical instruments and medical implements. The advance of the Greek physician was seen as a threat to this way of life.

Examples of Cato's prescriptions are found in his long section on the medicinal value of cabbage ('On Agriculture', CLVI-CLVIII). This is a vegetable which surpasses all others in usefulness, for Cato. 'It promotes digestion and is an excellent laxative, the urine [of the patient] is wholesome for everything.' Furthermore, 'If you wish to drink deep at a banquet and to enjoy your dinner, eat as much raw cabbage as you wish, seasoned with vinegar, before dinner, and likewise after dinner eat some half a dozen leaves; it will make you feel as if you had not dined, and you can drink as much as you please.' Cato states, 'Nothing will purge as well as wild cabbage, this the strongest cabbage.' He recommends that it should be dried and cut very fine; 'add oil, a very little salt, cumin, and fine barley-flour and let it boil very thoroughly'. This mixture should be eaten without bread, if possible; if the patient cannot do without bread, plain bread may be soaked in the mixture, and then, if the patient has no fever, he may have some dark wine. 'The cure will be prompt.' Cabbage was also good in a poultice for ulcers and fistulas, for suppurating wounds and tumours, for breast ulcers and cancer. It was equally good for painful hearts, and sore eyes, and, 'When all the veins in the whole body are gorged with food and they cannot breathe, if cabbage is eaten, no ill effects will ensue.'

Cato's list of medicines has a further interest. In the first place, his dietary advice is very close to, though somewhat simpler than, the Hippocratic treatise 'On Regimen'. Next, the idea of purgation as a means to good health, which was first noted in Egyptian and Greek culture, is also practised in Republican Rome. Furthermore, it is observed that the idea that veins carry blood and that arteries contain air, first found in early Egyptian medicine, and later in the philosphy of Alcmaeon of Croton (but disputed by Herophilus in Alexandria), remains unchanged in second-century BC Rome. Here Cato seems to confirm the findings of his predecessors. This is interesting, because Pliny has told us of Cato's great dislike of Greeks and Greek medicine (*Nat. Hist.* 39.7), a view which Pliny himself shared. Yet here, before Pliny's arrival on the scene, Cato is aware of some of the advantages of Greek methods and, perhaps unconsciously, using them in his own work. Varro, on the other hand, writing in the last years of the Roman Republic, compiled a similarly encyclopaedic handbook on farming to that of Cato, but he gives less attention to medical practices.

EARLY MEDICINE AT ROME

Although the rituals prescribed by Cato and Varro could not have cured a dislocated joint, or even the pain of gout, people would probably have found relief from their symptoms in much of this kind of therapy. Perhaps they would have found comfort in custom, in shared concepts and in the practices and triumphs of empiricism. In addition to these more positive features of ancient medicine the human body has a surprising facility to heal itself; many ills recover naturally, without too much interference. However, all this can only apply to the common complaints, such as colds, boils and sprains and summer diarrhoea. More complicated conditions, for example, disorders of the newly born, or severe medical and surgical problems, would have required specific help and perhaps surgery.

Childbirth would also have had its problems, even given the fact that in ancient times it was regarded as a natural function and not as an illness for which hospitalisation was necessary. Such an attitude may have made for easier childbirth in some fortunate cases, for others, in a few areas, physicians and possibly experienced midwives may have been available. Women would have had recourse to older women's advice regarding herbal medicine or amulets, in addition to religious medicine. Conversely, the lack of hygiene in this respect, and which prevailed in the West until the twentieth century, would have led to many maternal and infant deaths.

In some ways it is possible to regard the lack of special institutions, such as hospitals in which to care for the sick, as a positive feature of early medicine. In a community such as a modern hospital, treatment is occasionally hazardous. The sick are exposed to cross-infections and to the accidents of human error. Some diseases suffered by people in the past were the same as those of today; others were different – the plague of Athens, for example – or unknown in antiquity – AIDS, for instance.

URBANISATION AT ROME

To summarise the chapter so far, the above is an introduction to early Roman medicine. It has been demonstrated that, in the third-second centuries BC, this consisted of religion, folk medicine, magic and superstition. Nevertheless, with the passage of time and the influence of Greek culture, Roman medicine, both in theory and practice, was changing. Urbanisation was underway by the third century BC and people were no longer growing their own medicinal plants in rural areas. It became necessary for herbs to be transported to the towns, whether from the countryside or overseas. In the old cities and new towns living conditions were unhealthy. People suffered greatly from the use of unclean water, poor sanitation, malnutrition and overcrowding. Fires in the *insulae* were frequent, resulting in severe injuries or loss of life. Rome was in need of professional doctors. Although some Greek doctors had travelled to Rome earlier, these were not official appointments. The tradition is that Archagathus of Sparta, in 219 BC, was the first Greek doctor to enter Rome and to be appointed by the state (Pliny, *Nat. Hist.* 29.6.12-13). At first Archagathus was welcomed, he was given citizen's rights and a shop at the cross-way of Acilius. But, as a specialist in treating wounds, he was soon named 'Executioner' because of his savage use of the knife and cautery. As a result of this 'hiccup' in the state system, it seems that thereafter, all Greek physicians became objects of loathing. Pliny (*Nat. Hist.* 29.5.11) writes further:

> Hence those wretched, quarrelsome consultations at the bedside of the patient, no consultant agreeing with another lest he should appear to acknowledge a superior. Hence too that gloomy inscription on monuments: 'it was the crowd of physicians that killed me'. Medicine changes every day, being furbished up again and again, and we are swept along on the puffs of the clever brains of Greece,... just as if... people had not lived without physicians, though not without physic, as the Roman people have done for more than six hundred years.

Asclepiades (124-50 BC), from Bithynia (Rawson, 1982; but see Nutton 2004, 167, for a cogent discussion of his dates) in Asia Minor, on the other hand, was a more gentle and discerning doctor. He set up a practice in the late second century BC and captured aristocratic Rome with his irresistible slogan, 'softly, safely and sweetly' (*cito, tuto, jocunde*). From this it is seen that two Greek doctors gave the people of the Roman Republic entirely different experiences.

What was the experience of the Greek doctor seeking to practise his skills among Roman patients? Or of the Roman patient, recently arrived in a new town, from a rural area, who was forced to consult a Greek doctor? Changes and inequalities in today's health systems enable us to empathise with such a situation. In antiquity healers professed different systems and practised at various levels of knowledge and experience; this catered for all comers. By comparison, today's doctors are almost 'straitjacketed'. They are girded about by restrictions concerning the way they should do their work and how often they should see their patients, by chief executives and clinical managers, in order to meet targets within a system which, in many of its areas, is failing its patients. It is true, of course, that treatment available for patients is enormously improved and many therapies and medicines are almost miraculous in their effect, when compared with those of antiquity. However, at all the diverse levels of practice in ancient Rome, doctors, unlike those of today, could do very much as they considered best, and within that system patients had choices. The exception, of course, would have been the *medici* in the Roman Army who were subject to military supervision.

In Rome the integration of Greek and Roman medicine was lengthy and difficult. Although xenophobia, traditionalism and chauvinism played a part, these aspects are not the full story. Neither can the blame be put on the confrontation between Greek theory and Roman practicality, nor on the fact of urbanisation, or even Hellenisation. Although in many ways aristocratic Romans admired and emulated the Greeks in their art, fashion and personal styles, throughout the Republican period and beyond Greeks met with suspicion and dislike in other areas of life. This is particularly noticeable in medicine. Here Pliny (*Nat. Hist.* 29.8.19) reflects the thoughts of Cato:

> Medicine alone of the Greek arts we serious Romans have not yet practised; in spite of its great profits, only a few of our citizens have touched upon it, and even these at once were deserters to the Greeks.

It is possible that an explanation for Roman dislike of Greek physicians can be found elsewhere. A recent study examines the pre-existing cultural factors on both sides of the problem: just as a plurality of health-care systems was seen earlier, a plurality of cultural beliefs, backgrounds and expectations is also apparent. Healing works on different levels; Greek doctor and Roman patient, on first meeting, did not harmonise, they collided, resulting in 'fertile fields of misunderstandings'.[8] This 'clash of cultures' is reflected in the writings of contemporary Roman authors. The integration of Greek doctor and Roman patient was protracted and difficult because the Greek and the Roman came from different cultural backgrounds, with different knowledge and expections and beliefs; this would have been compounded by difficulties of communication and nomenclature. It is not known that Roman indigenous healing was ineffective, nor is it known that Greek science, or rationalism, guaranteed greater success. Eventually, however, with the coming of Galen (*c.*AD 129–216?) Greek and Roman attitudes began to coalesce.

HEALING WITH PLANTS

The healing powers of plants, their mind-altering effects and their analgesic properties have been exploited since earliest times. In Britain, in the Neolithic period, seeds of the plant *Hyoscimus niger*, or henbane (*23*), were found in a lump of carbonated porridge clinging to sherds of Grooved Ware pottery at a ritual centre at Balfarg in Fife.[9] It has already been shown that ceremonial use of the opium poppy (*24*) dates from at least as early as the thirteenth century BC. Poppy heads have a symbolic significance beyond their use as a food or drug. In the Greek world, poppies and wheatsheaves were attributes of Demeter, goddess of corn and agriculture. In the Roman world she was conflated with Ceres. In the Imperial period at Rome, poppy heads and stalks of grain are brought together in a lush landscape on the *Ara Pacis* (*25*), in a celebration of 'plenty' in childbearing and fecundity in nature. The purpose of this art is political. Although the availability of medicinal plants is known from art and literature, the way in which such drugs were used in antiquity is less well known.

EVIDENCE FOR MEDICINAL PLANTS ON COINS

When a plant is depicted on a coin, the purpose is, again, political and, as in the art-form discussed above, the illustration itself is evidence for the contemporary presence and use of that particular species. Additional informa-

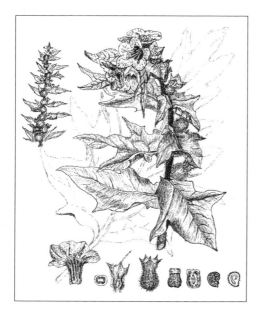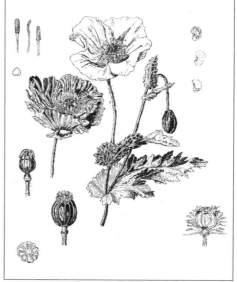

23 Left Henbane, *Hyoscyamus niger; 24 Right* The opium poppy, *Papaver somniferum*

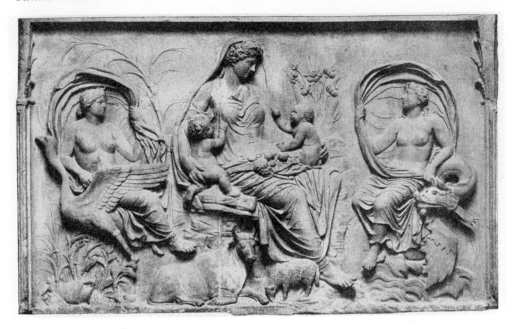

25 The Tellus relief on the *Ara Pacis*

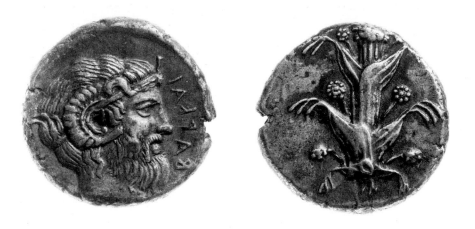

26 Greek coin of Cyrene, showing Zeus Ammon with a silphium plant on the reverse

tion is obtained from the date of the coin. The story of silphium is a case in point. Numismatic evidence suggests that the plant was familiar for centuries to countless numbers of people. Besides its use in seasoning food, it was employed in medicines and as an antiseptic. Writers ranging from Herodotus to Hippocrates, Theophrastus, Cato, Scribonius Largus, Dioscorides, Apicius (*fl. c.*AD 14–37) and Pliny all discussed knowledgeably the value of silphium. Other plants appearing on coins, both Greek and Roman, were the opium poppy, pomegranate, lily, wild celery and possibly hellebore.

Cyrene was a Greek city in North Africa. A full history of the founding of the colony is given by Herodotus (4.150-80). Evidence from Cyreniac coins demonstrates that silphium was produced and exported from 600-200 BC (*26*). Coins minted during this period have either the silphium fruit, leaf or whole plant engraved on them.[10] So valuable was silphium in the early period of the colony that it was regarded as a royal monopoly. Further affirmation of the importance of silphium to the economy of Cyrene is, perhaps, to be seen in the Arkesilas cup, painted in Sparta only some seventy years after the foundation of the colony[11] (*colour plate 11*).

The Romans valued silphium highly enough to have wanted to store it in the public treasury with the gold and silver. Theophrastus described the plant as having a thick root, a stalk like a ferula and a leaf like celery. It is identified as an umbellifer, probably the *Ferula tingitana*, which may be seen today in some botanical gardens. Pliny (*Nat. Hist.* 22.48.49) called the plant 'one of the most precious gifts of nature'; he cites many uses for silphium, of which a few are selected below:

> ...The leaves of silphium are used in medicine to purge the uterus and to bring away the still-born baby; a decoction of them is made in white, aromatic wine to be drunk after the bath in doses of one acetabulum. The root is good for soreness of the windpipe, and is applied to collections of extraversated blood... Laser, which is distilled from silphium, warms after chills... taken in drink it alleviates affections of the sinews. In wine it is given to women, and on soft wool is used as a pessary to promote menstruation. Mixed with wax it extracts corns from the feet... A piece the size of a chick-pea, diluted, is diuretic...

ANAESTHESIA AND PAIN RELIEF

In addition to a lack of knowledge concerning the needs and expectations of people in antiquity, it is also difficult to know whether pain was experienced in the same way as now, or whether it was regarded as something to be expected, a normal part of life which had to be 'put up with', or taken in one's stride.[12] It is possible, however, to say what medications would have been available, and to find out ways in which these may have been used. The henbanes (*Hyoscyamus niger* and *Hyoscyamus alba*) (*colour plate 12*) are members of the genus *Solanaceae*, the potato family. In this group of plants, several species possess pharmacological and psychotropic properties, and at least four of its members would have been useful in Roman surgery, namely datura or thorn-apple (*Datura stramonium*) (*colour plate 13*), mandrake (*Mandragora officiniarum*) (*colour plate 14*) and deadly nightshade (*Atropa belladonna*) (*colour plate 15*).

Later in history they became known as the 'saturnian herbs', because of their associations with witchcraft. Henbane, mandrake and datura possess a relaxant drug, hyoscine, from which scopolamine, used in modern anaesthesia, is made. Mandrake root, in modern anaesthesia, was the main anaesthetic before the development of ether. A rich folklore surrounded the gathering of the plant in the medieval period (*27*). Another psycho-active drug much valued in the ancient world was mugwort (*Artemisia vulgaris*, see chapter 6) (*colour plate 16*) which possesses hallucinogenic properties. However, most important was the opium poppy (*Papaver somniferum*); as a potent analgesic, it is today the source of morphine and heroin. Such was the variety of substances available in antiquity, quantities and compounds of which, mixed with wine, would have been very much down to trial and error. Regarding *Datura stramonium*, Theophrastus (*c.*371–*c.*287 BC, 'Enquiry', IX.II.6), writes: 'three-twentieths of an ounce in weight is given, if the patient is to become merely sportive and to think himself a fine fellow; twice this dose if he is to have delusions; thrice the dose if he is to be permanently insane; …four times the dose is to be given if he is to be killed'. Alternatively, Dioscorides states, '1 drachma [4 grams] in a drink is the quantity that allows one to have fantasies without unpleasantness, 2 drachmas alters one completely for three days, and 4 drachmas being drunk is fatal'.

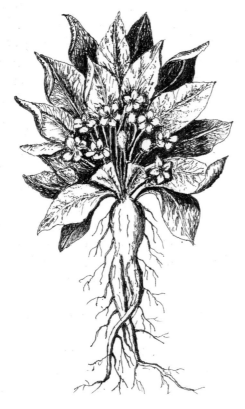

27 A copy of an eighteenth-century drawing of the 'magical' mandrake

All the drugs mentioned briefly above are extremely toxic, and the effects would vary according to the amount taken. Such drugs may have been easily available at markets and fairs, and at festivals too, as to some extent they are today. But, in contrast with the situation today, there were no checks or regulations governing their use. This was learned from experience, as well as instruction. Some physicians would have gained more knowledge and better skills than others and a few, perhaps, would have developed considerable expertise. Addiction could also have been a factor and, to some extent, this would account for the popularity of compounds of these drugs, such as the different theriacs that were available. Many of these theriacs contained opium in a mixture with wine, and are discussed further below.

According to Scarborough,[13] Hellenistic physicians were well aquainted with the dangers of opium poisoning; he suggests that Dioscorides stands in time on a bridge between Greek and Roman Imperial medicine. Moreover, Galen, according to Scarborough, repeats unchanged the findings on opium-producing poppies set down by Dioscorides.

Dioscorides of Anazarbus (*fl.* AD 70) practised medicine in southeastern Asia Minor. He may have studied botany and pharmacology in Tarsus, a city in which a collection of teachers in such subjects resided. His *De Materia Medica* appeared some time in the sixties or seventies of the first century and achieved instant popularity. It describes the uses of over 600 items, fused into 2,000 recipes and formulas. Embedded within his work, in modern times, a specific system has been discerned[14] in which Dioscorides' purpose seems to be to be to know 'what plants do'. This has been named the 'drug affinity system' by Scarborough and Riddle. In this system, Dioscorides, rather than demonstrating the form of the plant, centres his enquiry on the question of what happens when a patient is given a particular drug (or compound of drugs) in a particular ailment.

Dioscorides was much experienced in preparations of juice or latex from the opium poppy. In his account of its several uses he discusses benefits to the diet. He was aware that poppy-seeds have no narcotic properties but that they could be health-inducing (this has been confirmed by modern chemists who discovered lecithin in poppy-seed meal). It was possible to grow a weakened opium poppy in the garden for use in the diet either in bread, or as seeds sprinkled on the top of it, and for its oil, which was also nourishing. From this milder form of poppy-juice, decocted leaves and capsules applied to fomentations could be used to 'bring on sleep', or as a drink for insomnia. A mixture of pounded poppy capsules and hulled barley was used in a poultice, or it could be formed into cooling plasters for patients suffering from 'St Anthony's fire', erysipelas.

A further use for the mildly acting form of the drug was to make lozenges. This was achieved by pounding the leaves and mixing them with the decocted poppy capsules. Known as *trochisks*, the lozenges were laid out in the sun to dry and would have been easy to store and transport. A further advantage of this method was that they retained their medicinal properties and when reconstituted, were useful in plaster or in fomentations.[15] In addition Dioscorides prescribes stronger forms of opium for use as pain-killing lozenges for coughs and tracheal discharges, as well as for bowel conditions.

EYE SALVES

Oculists' stamps are used for making official impressions on sticks of dried, portable eye salves. These small objects are invaluable for their provision of at least three different types of primary evidence: pathological, pharmacological and archaeological. In this chapter it is the pharmacology which is of interest. The archaeology of collyrium stamps is discussed below in the chapter dealing with medical implements and surgical instruments.

Oculists' stamps bearing prescriptions for eye disease have been collected and recorded by scholars since the nineteenth century.[16] Included among the ingredients are saffron, gall and *glaucium*, which is either greater celandine or poppy (Pliny, *Nat. Hist*. 27.58-59). Eye salves were also made from copper oxide and 'misy'; the latter was copper pyrites (Pliny, *Nat. Hist*. 33). Wine would have been the chief ingredient contained in the vinegar salve. Other constituents included cinnabar, frankincense and myrrh. There was also an 'itch' salve made from balsam sap; the latter is alum and probably came from Melos. Pliny (*Nat. Hist*. 35. 187-8) writes that the best type is Milenum and comes from the island of Melos. The collyrium stamp (*RIB* 2446.9) found at Kenchester is inscribed '*Nardinum*, the salve of Ariovistus' (*colour plate 19*), a Celtic name; the salve is made from nard-oil. This is a precious and expensive substance belonging to the valerian plant family, which only could be obtained from the Eastern provinces. *Valerian officinalis*, however, is native to Britain. The alkaloids valerine and chatinine are present in this plant. It is used today as a sedative and tranquilliser, and also in the treatment of leprosy and cholera.

THE MICHIGAN MEDICAL CODEX, A LATE ROMAN PAPYRUS

Hippocratic physicians were already collecting therapeutic recipes in the fifth century BC and the Alexandrian period of medical development was also fertile in work on medicinal plants. However, the habit of naming a medicament after the physician or pharmacist from whose work it was taken, or with whom it was associated, only becomes frequent in the recipe collections of the Roman period. In the fourth century AD, a papyrus known as the 'Michigan Medical Codex'[17] has special relevance for the study of medicine in the Greek and Roman worlds. Although the context and provenance of the

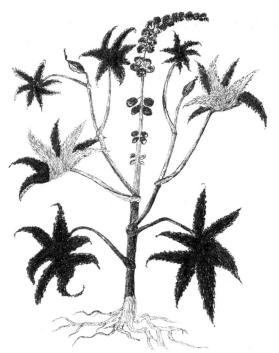

28 The castor-oil plant
(*Ricinus communis*), after
Dioscorides

codex is unknown – the papyrus was purchased from dealers in the 1920s – the contents indicate that the whole document was being put together and taking shape over a considerable period of time. The original owner was evidently a doctor who wrote down many recipes and who also employed a scribe. Two hands are discernible in the text, which may have been the lifetime's collection of a physician who had, at some time, access to a library. Many of the recipes were drawn from physicians and pharmacists who were practising in Rome early in the first century AD, such as Heras the Greek physician from Cappadocia, who practised in Rome *c*.20 BC-AD 20. Later recipes can be attributed to Galen and to Oribasius, physician to the Emperor Julian. The widespread and long-lasting nature of the recipes attests to their efficiency, and also to each prescription's integrity and completeness.

Within the codex are found recipes for pills and lozenges as well as for plasters, which can also be made into powders or dry applications by the omission of liquids. The main active ingredients are plants such as rue, willow, opium poppy and henbane, as well as metals, including malachite, copper flakes, scraped iron rust and lead monoxide. These are mixed with oils from different sources such as the castor-oil plant (*28*) rose, myrtle, myrrh, or crushed linseed. Animal fats are also used; these may be either 'weak' or 'strong'. Resin was another vital ingredient. It was obtained from pine, the juice of 'all-heal', valerian, and frankincense. The method of preparation for each prescription was carefully described.

In a discussion of ancient drug therapy, a number of important points need to be clarified. The Greek word *pharmaka*, which includes drugs, herbs, poisons, remedies and spells, is in itself an apt indicator of the empirical nature of ancient medicine, for the same word defines both medications and poisons. Examples are deadly nightshade and foxglove (*29*) which may either kill or cure, depending on the dose that is administered. Toxins are ubiquitous in plants and their power is more easily understood when it is realised that they have very specific and vital functions. Plants manufacture toxins for defence against predation by insects or other animals, as well as for protection from extremes of climate. Toxins are also the waste products of the plant's own metabolism. 'Pharmacognosy' is the scientific study of medicines and drugs that are derived from the natural world; 'pharmacology' is the science which both seeks to identify the interactions of drugs in the human body and to understand the attendant biochemical changes. Although modern medicine has the advantage of assistance from both of these disciplines, catastrophies nevertheless occur. How much more precarious was life in the ancient world where drugs were discovered by trial and error?

In addition to the caveats described above, the identification of ancient botanical terms is difficult and when it comes to correlating ancient and modern plant names, it cannot take it for granted that the names used in ancient times apply to similarly named plants in the modern botanical vocabulary. Although the Greeks and Romans laid the foundations for the method of naming plants and of observing and describing nature in detail,

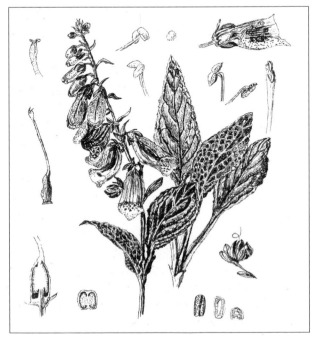

29 The foxglove, *Digitalis*

the binomial system in use today is largely due to the influence of Carl Linnaeus, who, in the eighteenth century, devised a different method for identifying plants from the descriptive method of the botanists and herbalists of ancient times.

> Not even the woods and the wilder face of Nature are without medicines, for there is no place where that holy Mother of all things did not distribute remedies for the healing of mankind, so that even the very desert was made a drug store, at every point occurring wonderful examples of that well-known antipathy and sympathy.
>
> Pliny, *Nat. Hist.* 24.1

Pliny praised the 'boundless grandeur of the *Pax Romana*' (*Nat. Hist.* 27.1) for making the empire the frame of a worldwide commerce in healing plants. One result of this was that many new species were introduced into Britain during the Roman period. Indeed, AD 43 is the benchmark recognised by botanists in Britain for determining whether a plant is native or introduced, though, of course, plants might have been introduced by merchants and travellers from the south for decades before this date. Further changes occurred to the flora of Britain and elsewhere when the great plant collectors brought new specimens from the Americas and Japan during the period from the sixteenth to the nineteenth centuries. In antiquity many of these lands had yet to be discovered. The age of hybrids, which began in the latter half of the twentieth century, brought about the generation of new plants, followed by the growth of nurseries. Today many modern plants and their names bear little resemblance to the plant names that were familiar to Theophrastus and those who followed him. This presents the historian of ancient pharmacy with difficulties.

However, in some cases Pliny's descriptions help to clarify the species that is being referred to. This source can be complemented by drawings appearing in surviving copies of a herbal which may have been the work illustrated by Crateuas, a botanist and root-cutter, who was physician to Mithridates VI, (120-63 BC) (Pliny, *Nat. Hist.* 25.4.8). He wrote a treatise on the nature and uses of herbs, but his most valued work is his second herbal, in which plants were illustrated. Dioscorides' herbal, written in Greek, was the result of a lifetime's study. Its layout was systematic with detailed observation combined with a rejection of superstition and magic and was later approved by Galen. The *Codex Vindobonensis Medicus Graecus*, popularly known as the 'Vienna Dioscorides' (also known as the 'Juliana Anicia Codex') was made in Constantinople in 512 for Princess Anicia Juliana, the daughter of the Western Roman Emperor Anicius Olybrius.[18] The manuscript is well illustrated with drawings and text, including descriptions and uses of plants and paintings of insects, reptiles and arachnids, and also drawings of twenty-four birds. On one

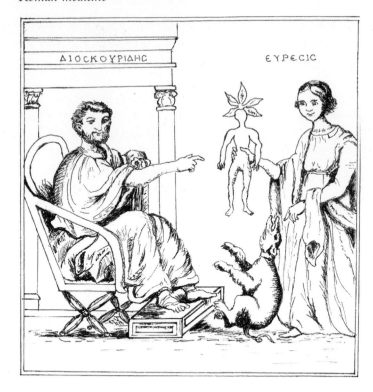

ΔIOCΚΟΥΡΙΔΗC   ΕΥΡΕCΙC

30 Dioscorides receives from the hand of Euresis, goddess of discovery, the mandrake root with its magical powers; the dog died during its uprooting. *Copied from a restoration drawing in the 'Codex Vindobonensis' of Dioscorides in the National Library, Vienna*

page is a portrait, possibly of Dioscorides seated and writing in a book, whilst an artist, thought to be Crateuas, makes a drawing of a mandrake (*30*). The drawings in the 'Vienna Dioscorides' may be derived from those of Crateuas. He was consulted widely.[19]

In modern times, an invaluable source is found in a new study[20] centred on both ancient and modern Pompeii. It is written by Wilhelmina Jashemski, a scholar and archaeologist, who has also worked on and written about the archaeology of the gardens of Pompeii. Archaeological evidence, primary written sources and the observations and learning of modern, native gardeners and workmen, combine to provide an authentic example of the continuity of life in the shadow of Mount Vesuvius. In addition to this publication, a significant study of plant remains from the site of Pompeii itself is of interest (*31*).

A PHARMACY IN THE ITALIAN COUNTRYSIDE?

Although all conclusions drawn from archaeological evidence are to be treated with caution, the following investigation is pertinent to the present theme of the book. In 1996, the excavation of a farmhouse,[21] *villa rustica*, near Pompeii, uncovered seven storage vats, *dolia*, in a cellar. They contained deposits rich

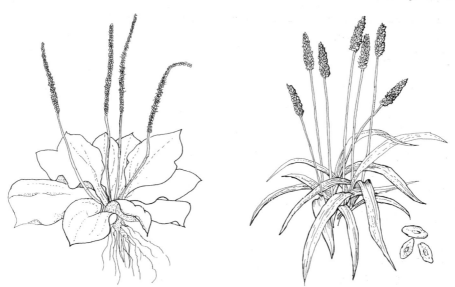

31 Left a) Psyllium *(Plantago ovata)* with three of its unhusked seeds enlarged; *Right* b) *Plantago major L.;* this is used at Pompeii to treat colitis. Both types of plantain were used in antiquity. Both Pliny *(Nat. Hist.* 25.80) and Dioscorides (2.153), amongst other ancient authors, write of the medicinal benefits to be obtained from these plants

in seeds of plants known for their use in medicines and in mixtures such as mithridatum and theriac. Bones of reptiles and amphibians were also present. Organic deposits from the bottom of all seven *dolia* were found to be water-logged, therefore the sample for analysis, taken from *dolium* 2, came from a perfectly sealed context. The villa had been covered by several metres of lapilli, similar in depth to those which overlay the town of Pompeii itself, and evidently from the same eruption of the volcano. 'Villa Vesuvio' was therefore firmly dated to AD 79. Some of the plants identified in these organic remains include those with medical properties known to have been in continuous use for many thousands of years. References to them are found in Egyptian and Greek medicine and also in the writings of Pliny, Dioscorides and Scribonius Largus.

Among other plant remains were opium poppy, also members of the *gens solanaceae: Symphytum officiale* L., comfrey, and *Cannabis sativa* L., hemp. Large quantities of unripe *Punica granatum* L., pomegranate, were discovered here, too. The plant was praised by several authors: Cato ('On Agriculture', CXXVII), gives a recipe for strangury and dyspepsia using blossoms of pomegranate *(colour plate 20)*. Celsus describes a variety of uses for the fruit, usually in combination with other ingredients, ranging from pain relief to treatment for ear infections. Dioscorides, too, mentions uses for pomegranate and Pliny discusses the fruit at some length. Hippocrates, Soranus and Aetius prescribe the seeds and rind of the plant for use as a contraceptive.[22]

Inside the villa was an open space which the excavators interpreted as a threshing floor, a wine press, *torcularium*, and an associated cellar, *cella vinaria*. The cellar contained the *dolia*, which were visible as large vats partly embedded in the ground. A particular type of small cooker was also present. Similar cookers have been found at other sites in and around Pompeii; two were observed in medical workshops from which surgical instruments were also recovered. A similar oven was also found at the *villa rustica* of L. Crassus Tertius, outside the city walls at Oplontis. The ovens are especially interesting when considered together with the scene represented on a Roman votive stele, found in southern France, now kept at the Grand Museum of Epinal[23] (*colour plate 21*). According to the researcher, this portrays exactly the type of cooker found in the Villa Vesuvio and in the houses in and around Pompeii, described above. The scene depicted in the bas-relief is generally believed to represent a pharmacy or soap manufactory.

The *villa rustica* at Oplontis, in addition to the pomegranates and oven found there, produced several metres of carbonised hay. Archaeologists discovered that the hay was originally collected from a nearby vineyard and transported to the villa. As a result of this find, after scientific analysis, fresh information was forthcoming concerning the flora present in the area at the time of the volcanic eruption. So far, 128 new taxonomic species have been identified in the hay. These include carbonised blossoms, seeds, leaf and stem fragments, and the pollen of many wild flowers and weeds. All have been added to the archaeobotanical plant record.

THERIAC AND MITHRIDATE

In first-century AD Pompeii, a pharmacy in the Italian countryside would have been an ideal situation for a family business manufacturing medications such as theriac. A wide variety of flora would have been available in the area. Mithridate and theriac have an interesting history. Mithridates, King of Pontus (132-63 BC), was a savage tyrant and an inveterate enemy of Rome and, like many such bullies, he lived in fear for his life. Most of all he was afraid he would be poisoned (Celsus, *De Med.* V.23.2-4; Pliny, XXIX,23-26). He studied the subject of poison and concocted the idea that a little of a certain mixture taken each day would cause him to become so used to it that a large amount of the substance taken inadvertently would not kill him. The king thus became immune to poisons. Eventually, wanting to take his own life, he found poison to be ineffective and was forced to die by the sword with his own hand. His recipes were collected by Pompey, who was also interested in antidotes to poisons. By this time poisoning was becoming an accepted risk to life at Rome.

Theriac, on the other hand, was originally devised for bites, of either human or animal origin. According to Pliny (*Nat. Hist.* 28.39) 'The bite of a human being is considered to be a most serious one', whilst those from wild animals were especially to be feared where Roman armies fought in distant and hostile territories. After Mithridates the recipes became more complex until, at times, more than sixty-four compounds could be involved, causing Pliny to complain, 'Which of the gods, in the name of Truth, fixed these absurd proportions?' Indeed, Galen devoted an entire book to the subject, called *Theriake*. Theriacs became extremely popular and the Roman traveller regarded his theriac in much the same way as vaccination is thought of today.[24] However, the effect of a theriac was more that of comfort and a placebo than proper medication.

ROMAN HERB GARDENS

Although both Theophrastus and Lucretius are known to have possessed gardens (*horti*) these have not been found archaeologically. Gardens as such were not generally known before they were developed by the Romans who would grow medicinal plants, flowers, fruit and vegetables in them. Pliny tells us (*Nat. Hist.* 25.9):

> I at least have enjoyed the good fortune to examine all but a very few plants through the devotion to science of Antonius Castor, the highest botanical authority of our time; I used to visit his special garden, in which he would rear a great number of specimens even when he had passed his hundredth year, having suffered no bodily ailment and, in spite of his age, no loss of memory or physical vigour.

Roman gardens often evolved as extensions to the house, for dining in areas shaded by pergolas and ornamented colonnades, usually embellished with water features. Use was made of portable furniture such as tables and couches and the ambience would have been one of relaxation. Such a house as this would also possess baths and possibly a gymnasium. Thus the concepts for good health required by the Hippocratic treatise 'On Regimen' would have been observed in the houses of the elite. On the other hand, 'Trimalchio's dinner-party'[25] demonstrates, with great humour, the extremes of overeating and *luxuria* which were possible.

ROMAN BRITAIN

The Druids, perhaps best regarded as a priestly caste, were evidently the most learned amongst the native population. However, little reliable evidence is available concerning them, or their ways of healing. A variety of native plant species would have been useful for herbal cures: for example, *Glechoma hedera* (ground ivy), *Angelica sylvestris* (wild angelica), *Nepeta cataria* (catmint), *Malva/ Althaea sp.* (marshmallow), *Peucedanum officianale* (dill), *Myra gale* (wax myrtle), *ruta graveolens* (rue, 'herb of grace'), *and Verbena officianalis* (vervain). Other plants such as the *Solanaceae* would also have been available. *Linum* (flax) is known from a few sites, and Celsus (*De Med.* V.26 and 23) informs us that it makes good bandages. It is, of course, useful for making clothes, too. A degree of knowledge is attested in the use of mistletoe, *Viscaceae album*, which, as Pliny (*Nat. Hist.* 16.95) tells us, the Druids regarded as sacred. Mistletoe was found among the stomach contents of 'Lindow man' (Turner and Scaife, 1995). The plant has compounds which affect the heart and circulatory system, and, perhaps because of these magical properties, there may also have been attempts to use it therapeutically.

In Britain, in addition to native folk medicine, the Roman Army may have imported dried herbs for immediate use and storage, as well as introducing new varieties of seeds. Foreign plants and herbs are known from environmental archaeology to have entered the archaeo-botanical record early in the Roman period.[26] Weeds were introduced with crops by Roman, or even earlier, agriculturalists. It is probable that the opium poppy was amongst them, for the presence of the plant has been recorded from at least twenty archaeological sites. However, it may not have been possible to extract opium from the poppies grown in Roman Britain, due to the climate which prevailed at that time.

ROMAN INFLUENCE IN BRITAIN

Romans developed the art of wine-making and they brought the grape and the art of viticulture to Britain.[27] Wine was often used as a vehicle for medication and medicated wine was exported in amphorae throughout the empire. A sherd of such an amphora, which had possibly contained medicinal wine, was sent to the vexillation fortress at Carpow, in Britain, in the early third century,[28] the inscription πρασι [ον], 'horehound', is read with some difficulty. Dioscorides gives a prescription for a wine flavoured with horehound, or *prasion*, to treat chest complaints and coughs (*De Med.* XLVIII). Celsus and Pliny also recommend horehound for treating these ailments. At Caerleon, too, an amphora with the graffito AMINE, 'Aminean' wine, is found.[29] This medication was a kind of 'cure-all', devised for the treatment of diarrhoea and also for the common cold (*De Med.* IV.5.2; IV.26.3.9).

At Fishbourne Roman Palace, near Chichester, the formal garden of a large villa or palace, probably the residence of the client king Tiberius Claudius Togidubnus, was first excavated in the 1960s and has now been restored.

Many later villas had extensive gardens and gardens were also to be found in town houses. Although in many instances formal plantings with decorative shrubs and flowers or fruit trees and the like were grown, it is likely that, as in much later monastic gardens, such green spaces supplied the pharmacopoeia as well, and although in the past insufficient attention has been paid to this aspect of Roman life, hopefully there will be more organised attempts to extract such evidence in the future. Some idea of what a Roman medicinal garden might have looked like is shown at Fishbourne in a bed planted with a variety of herbs. Even formal gardens could have been used. For the most part the reconstructed palace garden at Fishbourne seems too bland. There would, perhaps, have been more variety in the plants employed around the edgings and to judge from the great garden painting from Livia's villa at Prima Porta (end of the first century BC) the grass would not have been kept short but would have had more of the appearance of a flower meadow. These plants would in many instances have been harvested for medicinal use – a good example of Roman pragmatism in blending practicality with beauty.

~ 4 ~

ROMAN HEALTH AND HYGIENE
THE BUILDINGS

The Romans had the best foresight in those matters of which the
Greeks made but little account, such as the construction of roads,
aqueducts and sewers.

Strabo, *Geog.*, 5.3.8[1]

Although Greek culture developed earlier than that of the Romans, the
Romans were not without their independent native refinements and
their artistic and intellectual achievements. Strabo (64 BC–after AD 24), was a
Greek geographer who, visiting Rome in 44 BC at the age of twenty, as part
of his education, developed a profound admiration for Roman culture. Even
today, it is possible to find sufficient primary evidence, both archaeological and
written, in support of the engineering and building achievements of ancient
Romans.

As well as roads, aqueducts and sewers, many of which still remain in use,
there were baths, both public and private, the drainage of disease-harbouring
marshlands and a fire service. All these were instigated by Roman politicians
and designed by Roman engineers. Such innovations would have provided for
a healthier and safer way of life at every level of society. Furthermore, for the
Roman Army, there possibly were purpose-built hospitals.

In general, the development of Roman engineering owed much to influences gained from other peoples. In particular, such progress was assisted by
Greek engineers working for Romans. This led to the diffusion of ideas and
practices. Yet, Roman engineers, already possessed of innate technical virtu-
osity, took engineering much further and eventually Rome's water supply was
rendered unique by the sheer size of its supply system. This public utility was
provided in cities and towns throughout the empire.

WATER SUPPLY

The most basic requirement for good health and human survival is a suffi-
ciency of clean water. Rome's water supply has been widely researched by
archaeologists and classical historians and although there is more to learn,
much of the system is already well understood. Books written in both ancient
and modern times are available on the subject.[2] According to Cicero, the
credit for the original selection of the site of Rome was given to Romulus for
his observation of the many rising natural water-sources (*Rep.* 2.6.11). Pliny,
on the other hand, comments on the wonders of the natural water supply:
…'this element is lord over all others…'; (*Nat. Hist.* 31.1). Pliny also writes,
'Everywhere in many lands gush forth beneficent waters, here cold, there
hot, there both' (*Nat. Hist.* 31.11.1). For several centuries Rome's natural
supplies, the abundant springs and local wells, appear to have been adequate
to meet demands. Water could also have been taken directly from the River
Tiber. Yet by the fourth century BC, increasing urbanisation was affecting
these sources and the amount of water obtained from them was neither
sufficient nor suitable to meet the needs of the city's ever-expanding population. Efforts were already underway to bring water into Rome from outside
the city by aqueduct. However, water is easily contaminated. Furthermore,
given contemporary social conditions as well as an absence of knowledge
concerning infection, such contamination would have been all too easily
spread throughout communities. Thus life-giving water could also be a source
of death-dealing infections and the water-supply of Rome was extremely
vulnerable to such pollution.

The earliest aqueducts to supply Rome were the Aqua Appia, built in
312 BC and the Aqua Anio Vetus, in 272 BC. They were not carried on
arches, but passed through underground channels (*specus* or *rivi*) which were
cheaper to construct and which kept the water safe from Rome's enemies.
At the same time, this type of design acted as a necessary safeguard from theft
and also from possible contamination. The Aqua Appia was about 16.5km in
length, even though its sources were only 11km from Rome. The disparity
was due to the complication of following the contours of the land. The Aqua
Marcia, built in 144 BC, was the first Roman aqueduct to be carried partly
on bridges, alternating with the traditional tunnels. Unlike the high-pressure
water systems of modern times, which are connected to taps in private houses,
the earliest Roman system was designed to produce a constant gravitational
flow for use by the general public. The water would be collected from central
points, such as the street fountains (*salientes*) and public basins (*lacus*). Public
and private baths (*balneae*) were also supplied by aqueducts and the perpetual
overflow produced by the fountains and the baths was utilised in the constant
sewer flushing (Frontinus, *De Aquis Urbis Romae* Bk 2.111). This is a water-
conserving device which modern systems would do well to emulate.

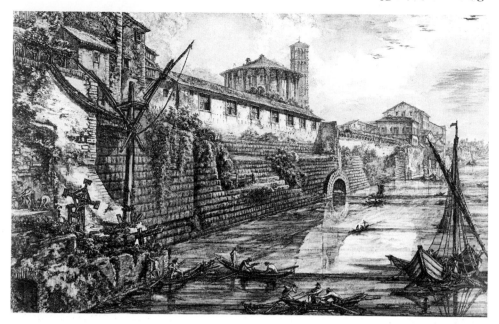

32 Piranesi's etching, 'The Tiber at the mouth of the Cloaca Maxima'

As aedile in 33 BC, Marcus Agrippa (64-12 BC) concerned himself with the water supply and sewage system of Rome (*32*). During the late Republic the city fathers, either impoverished or else reluctant to spend money, had allowed needs to become urgent before introducing new aqueducts. Therefore, there was much work to be done. Agrippa's remedies were extensive, designed to meet the needs of the Augustan building programme. He revolutionised the city's water system. At his own expense, he repaired the old aqueducts Appia, Anio Vetus and Marcia and constructed a new aqueduct, the Aqua Julia. This helped to supplement and to improve the quality of the warmish water of the smaller Aqua Tepula. Agrippa's major single personal donation to Rome, however, was the construction of the Aqua Virgo in 20 BC. This was brought in from the north to serve the Campus Martius and the Transtiber. The generous supply of water which came from this aqueduct allowed Agrippa to make his new public baths in the Campus Martius fully operational, thus giving to the people of Rome the first Imperial heated baths (*thermae*). The final plans for his great baths buildings were laid out in 20 BC, close to where the Pantheon now lies. Little of them survives. Today the water feeds the famous Trevi fountain, which of course belongs to a much later period in history. It was Agrippa's generous increase in the number of fountains in his day that made Rome's water supply so abundant and readily available to the people. Besides his work on the aqueducts, according to Pliny (*Nat. Hist.* 31.42), Agrippa built no fewer than 700 basins, 500 fountains and 130 distribution points or water towers (*castella*), from which water was delivered to Rome's private citizens' houses (*privatae domus*) and to the public cisterns. The amounts of water carried to the city are difficult to quantify but the actual volume may have been virtually doubled.

After the death of Agrippa in 11 BC, Imperial administration of the water system became firmly established with the creation of the office of Water Commissioner (*curator aquarum*). This was a prestigious appointment, and the custodian of such a position carried a great weight of personal responsibility. Agrippa's schedule and the planning (*commentarii*) that regulated it became the foundation for this new post.[3] Augustus' expansion of the boundaries of Rome had increased the size of the city, resulting in the need for a further aqueduct, the Aqua Augusta. Gaius Caesar began two more aqueducts; these were completed by Claudius. By AD 38 and AD 42 respectively the Aqua Claudia and the Anio Novus were in use. They entered the city at a higher level than the earlier aqueducts and were thus able to mete out water to its every region. Even after the death of Augustus in AD 14, the city of Rome was not entirely dependent on aqueducts for its water. As already noted, the site was naturally well watered by springs and due to the high water-table at Rome it could easily be drawn from hand-dug wells.[4] Water from the Tiber, too, was freely available and could be collected and stored in household cisterns. However, the sewage and detritus from the whole population of the city continually emptied into the river. This included the corpses of human beings and animals, as well as waste products from the tanneries which existed along the Tiber bank. The unsuitability of this water for drinking is evident, even when given the possibility that there could have been a degree of immunity amongst those who were accustomed to it. Once collected, the water would have been especially dangerous if stored in conditions where bacteria could thrive and multiply, such as in domestic cisterns, or barrels, which perhaps were left standing in the sun for uncertain lengths of time.

Vitruvius Pollio, a Roman architect and military engineer, (*c.*50-26 BC) composed a treatise, *De Architectura*, divided into ten books of which the eighth was concerned with water supply. Vitruvius (*De Arch.* 8.6.1-2) described the way that water, delivered to towns by aqueducts, was distributed:

> There are three methods of conducting water, in channels through masonry conduits, or in pipes made of lead or baked clay. If in conduits, let the masonry be as solid as possible, and let the bed of the channel have a gradient of not less than a quarter of an inch for every hundred feet, and let the masonry structure be arched over, so that the sun may not strike the water at all. When the water has reached the city, build a reservoir with a distribution tank in three compartments connected with the reservoir to receive the water, and let the reservoir have three pipes, one for each of the connecting tanks, so that when the water runs over from the tanks at the ends, it may run into the

one between them. From this central tank, pipes will be laid to all the basins and fountains; from the second tank, to baths, so that they may yield an annual income to the state; and from the third, to private houses, so that water for public use will not run short; for people will be unable to divert it if they have only their supplies from headquarters. This is the reason why I have made these divisions, and also in order that individuals who take water into their houses may by their taxes help to maintain the conducting of the water by the contractors.[5]

Vitruvius recommended earthenware pipes (*De Arch.* 8.6.10). Concerning these, he writes: 'water is much more wholesome when delivered in earthenware pipes than it is when lead pipes are used, for it seems to be made injurious by lead, because white lead is produced by it and this is said to be harmful to the human body'. The subject of lead poisoning in the Roman Empire is one of continuing debate and is discussed more fully below. Yet, despite the learned advice of Vitruvius, because it was both malleable and relatively inexpensive, lead continued to be used for domestic water pipes – and much else besides, including the manufacture, storage and serving of wine (*33*).

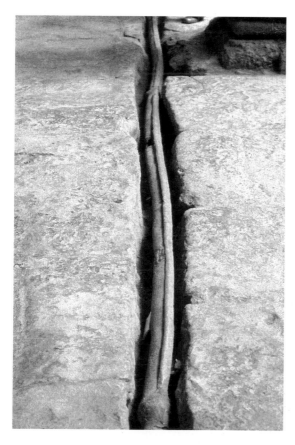

33 Roman Bath, a lead water-pipe

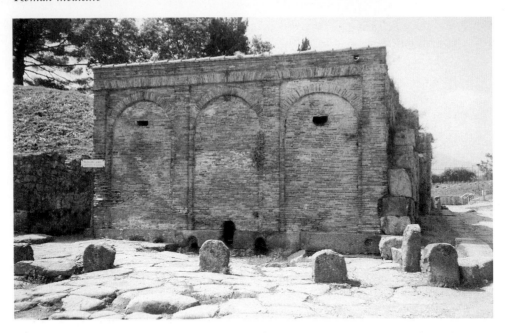

34 A *castellum aquarum* at Pompeii

In connection with the theme of water supply, names other than Marcus Agrippa and Vitruvius Pollio are important, especially that of Sextus Julius Frontinus (*c*.AD 30-*c*.104). After a successful governorship of Britain (*c*.AD 74-78) he was appointed *curator aquarum* of the Roman water supply in AD 97 by the Emperor Nerva. He subsequently wrote a work on the water supply of Rome, *De Aquis Urbis Romae*, in two books. On taking office, Frontinus encountered fraud, illegal taps, and theft of water from open channels; there were severe structural failures, too. All these factors caused a serious depletion in Rome's water supply. More than any other of his endeavours, Frontinus' efforts were directed towards putting an end to corruption. In addition to this undertaking, he worked hard to improve the aqueduct system itself and it was due to measures instigated by him that Rome's water supply again almost doubled. Because no water was improperly diverted, a sufficient supply was available for personal, domestic and municipal use. The city's appearance was cleaner, the air was purer and the previously unhealthy atmosphere lifted (*De Aquis.* 11.88). Doubtless, this was also largely due to the improved facilities for public bathing. Frontinus' supervision of the repairs of aqueducts and his rooting-out of law-breakers, enabled Rome's technical achievements to be fully restored. Indeed, such was Frontinus' pride in his improvements to the city, that he was tempted into saying, 'With such an array of indispensable structures carrying so many waters, compare, if you will, the idle Pyramids of Egypt or the useless, though famous, works of the Greeks!' (*De Aquis.* 1.16).[6] Conclusions, surely, with which, if we are honest, we would have agreed.

As vital as the provision of an adequate quantity of water was the question of its quality and its purity (*34*). This varied according to the source and method of delivery. In antiquity, of course, the standards applied to assess water were rudimentary; they mainly took account of such obvious factors as taste, smell, temperature and appearance. The Aqua Anio Novus, for example, whose source was the River Anio which could become muddy after storms, was reserved, according to Frontinus (*De Aquis.* Bk II.90-92) for industrial use and irrigation. The Marcia provided much better drinking water. Nevertheless, even when it reached the consumer, the purity of the piped water could not be vouched for. On the other hand Frontinus did not disparage the use of water from natural springs, for he informs us that some of them possessed beneficial curative powers (*De Aquis.* Bk I.4) and that many were associated with healing sanctuaries (discussed in chapter 5). Frontinus estimated that by his day 44 per cent of the total delivery of water was piped to private houses. He described the aqueducts and their history, the strict laws and regulations which governed them, and other technical details.

To remove impurities and to aerate the water, it was passed through numbers of settling tanks, *piscinae*. These were incorporated along the line, between the source and the distribution tanks. Not only would this practice return the sparkle to the water, it would also improve its flavour and, thus restored, it would be more healthy to drink. Frontinus was well aware of the benefits to life and health of plentiful supplies of clean water; he cites both 'public needs and private pleasures' (*De Aquis.* Bk I. 22-24) as the reasons for the introduction of the Claudian lines. However, Frontinus did not live to see the building of the last great aqueduct, the Aqua Traiana. This carried high-quality water to the Transtiber. A Trajanic inscription[7] cites its completion on 24 June, AD 109. By the end of the first century AD, Rome was supplied with nine aqueducts. Approximately a third of the water was distributed outside the city to suburban villas where it would have been used for the irrigation of farms and gardens as well as domestic purposes. Imperial properties outside the city also received part of the suburban distribution. It is notable that the largest concentration of suburban villas nearer to Rome is found along the route taken by the Anio Vetus, Marcia, Tepula and Julia and along the line of the Aqua Claudia into the city.[8]

From the time of Augustus onwards, the inhabitants of Rome undoubtedly received adequate water for all their necessities. It is possible that the history of the construction of aqueducts demonstrates that these were built in response to the needs of an expanding population. Much less certain, however, was the quality and purity of the water, especially where it was received at public basins by the homeless and by the bulk of the population who could not afford to have water piped to their dwellings. Pollution was liable to occur in any number of ways from the water's source to its delivery, from the use of contaminated containers for carrying water to casual refuse disposal beside supply lines. Contamination might also occur from people using public basins with unclean hands, to 'squatting' beside open water channels.[9] Basins and fountains were traditionally a focus for socialisation, so the potential for water contamination was ever-present. Partial knowledge of the possibility that water pollution could cause disease is perhaps evidenced by its being a punishable offence to contaminate the public water supply. An inscription prohibiting the pollution of water with excrement found above a water basin at Pompeii, demonstrates that such behaviour was a possibility.[10] Those who drank water from public water basins would have been more at risk from water-borne diseases than the villa owners whose water was piped into their homes from covered distribution tanks. At Pompeii, Rome and towns and cities elsewhere, both graffiti and literary evidence[11] demonstrate that people relieved themselves in streets and doorways, on tombs and behind statues. This would have applied especially to the *insulae* at Rome, Pompeii or Ostia where the blocks of dwellings did not possess a ground-floor latrine.

What diseases could be caused by water pollution? The most common gastro-intestinal infections are cholera, typhoid, dysentery and infective hepatitis. Contaminated water may also cause helminths – dangerous intestinal parasitic diseases such as threadworm, tapeworm, guinea-worm, whipworm and roundworm. In addition, diseases such as salmonella are carried by blow-flies and their pupae and these also contaminate standing water. Lucian writes in his panegyric of that small insect with its unpleasant habits:[12] 'flies are born of maggots from the dead bodies of humans or animals and live on the same food and eat at the same table as man'. The verse not only illuminates the havoc that can be wrought by a mere fly as it follows its natural life-cycle, it also demonstrates that some people were not entirely ignorant of the dangers of this type of contamination, even though in most situations avoidance would have been impossible. The slightest contact of an object with human or animal manure provides the fly with a perfect breeding ground. Diarrhoea is mentioned frequently in the literary sources[13] and would have been a constant scourge, causing fatality in the aged, in women who were 'lying-in' and in newly-born infants. In such cases, where there was already low immunity and, because the mode of transmission was ill understood, the weakest members of society would have found these infections impossible to withstand.

WATER SUPPLY ELSEWHERE IN THE EMPIRE

Municipal authorities initiated aqueduct construction and the system employed in Roman towns emulated in many ways the paradigm set by Rome. In modern times the physical remains of magnificent aqueducts can still be seen throughout the former territories of the Roman Empire, such as those at the Pont du Gard in France, and at Segovia and Toledo in Spain. Further examples are found at Aspendus in Turkey (*35, 36, 37*) and in Tunis in North Africa. In

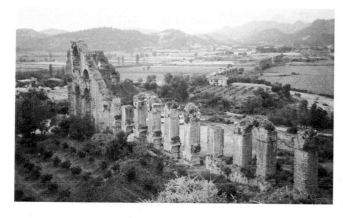

35 The aqueduct at Aspendus in Turkey

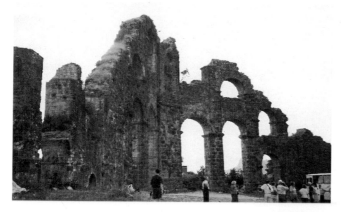

36 The arches of the aqueduct at Aspendus

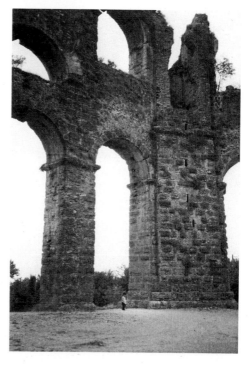

37 The columns of the aqueduct at Aspendus, demonstrating its great height

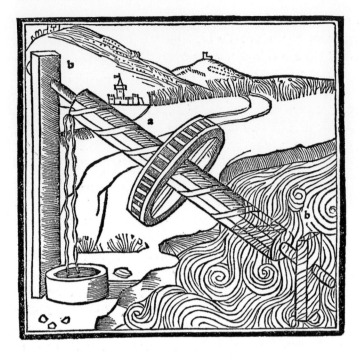

38 Vitruvius' water screw.
From the edition of Vitruvius by Fra Giocondo, Venice, 1511

Roman Britain aqueducts are known at York, Lincoln, Wroxeter, Dorchester in Dorset[14] and Leicester, although, as at Rome, other forms of water-supply systems were also employed.

Descriptions of a variety of water-lifting machinery (*38*) are found in Vitruvius (*De Arch.* 10.5-7). In addition, examples of such machinery recently discovered in Gresham Street in London are described and illustrated in *Current Archaeology* (180, pp.509-16). In Roman London more than a hundred wells have been excavated. Elsewhere in Britain, where wells are frequently found on Roman sites, old wine-barrels are often used for well-liners, as seen at the Roman town of Silchester (*Calleva Atrebatum*), in Hampshire.[15] However, wells in Roman towns were all too frequently positioned near cesspits or rubbish-tips, which is a further indication that there was generally minimal understanding of water-contamination as a cause of disease. Rain-water was often collected in barrels as well as in the *impluvia* of villas. It was valued more for its reputation of being 'soft' than for any quality of cleanliness and was recommended for diluting compounds of medications in the treatment of diarrhoea[16] and also for letting down collyrium from sticks of eye salve.

DRAINS AND SEWERS

Water supply and baths are not the only contributions to public health for which Marcus Agrippa should be given credit. He was also responsible for reconstructing the sewers so that they worked properly. The main sewer of Rome was the Cloaca Maxima, whose earliest construction is attributed to the Etruscan King Tarquinius Superbus in the late sixth century BC. It was originally an open watercourse which carried waters from the Esquiline, Viminal, and Quirinal hills to the Tiber, via the marshes of the Forum Romanum. Sometime in the third century BC, the massive sewer was enclosed. It is probable that ventilation to the sewer was provided by perforated manhole covers, as indicated by Suetonius (*De Gramm. et Rhet. 2*), who provides the information that sometime in the second century BC the maths master and *grammaticus*, Crates of Mallos in Cilicia, fell into the sewer through a manhole cover in the Palatine, breaking his leg, which forced him to prolong his stay in Rome. Later, as a result of Agrippa's work, the marshland became sufficiently drained to allow large-scale building on the site. In the year 33 BC, at the same time as he was working on Rome's water supply, Agrippa implemented the vaulting and paving of the Cloaca Maxima. The rebuilt mouth of the great sewer, still visible within the modern embankment, is probably his work. It remains part of the drainage system of the modern city of Rome. Agrippa cleaned out and repaired Rome's sewer networks (Suetonius *Aug.* 30) and is reputed to have sailed through part of them by boat into the Tiber (Pliny, *Nat. Hist.* 36.24.103-6).

All this time, while sewer connections had no traps, explosions of hydrogen sulphide and methane gases could occur inside people's homes, causing dangerous and unpleasant odours. They were also a potential cause of fire. However, this was not the only consequence to follow from the lack of traps.[17] In Rome the sewers in low-lying areas could back up when the level of water in the Tiber rose. Sewage and waste water, instead of flowing into the river by way of the Cloaca Maxima, or some other sewer, would be forced to return into the network and waste water and effluent could then have been driven back into house connections. Even without the danger of backwash, the untrapped drain connection between basin and sewer was a hazard to health. In addition, it was possible for vermin in the sewers to enter homes through any of the sewer pipework. Scobie cites an anecdote in Aelian[18] where 'an octopus swims up a house-drain each night from the sea to eat pickled fish stored in the house by Iberian merchants'.

Much more unpleasant would have been odours caused by the storage and collection of the urine which stood in jars in Roman towns and cities. Besides being unglazed and porous, the jars would often crack and burst, thus spilling their foul-smelling contents onto the streets. The urine was collected to be used by tanners; it was also required by fullers for mordanting dyestuffs and for stiffening cloths. Indeed, the Emperor Vespasian imposed a tax on the enterprise, thus indicating the scale of the business. This area of commerce was no less unpleasant than the collection and sale of human manure, by those who emptied cesspits (*stercorarii*) to farmers on city outskirts for agricultural purposes.[19] Possible dangers to the health of people who engaged in such trades are easy to imagine. At Pompeii, latrines in some houses had drains which led directly into the garden, thus contributing further to the noisome atmosphere.

LATRINES

Roman lavatories were similar to those that we are accustomed to find in Western Europe or the eastern Mediterranean in modern times, *ie*. the sit-upon type. Some lavatory seats were simply flat pieces of wood with a hole, whilst others, such as the public latrine (*forica*) at Ostia and Ephesus, had seats of marble (*39*). It is not known whether they were for single-sex or mixed use. In other cultures and parts of the world, in both ancient and modern times, the squatting position is adopted over a deep-dug hole in the ground the cover of which may, or may not, be substantially built, as encountered in Sudan. The latrine may also consist of a hole in the floor of a bathroom on an upper storey of a house. In this case a chute would be built through which waste material could fall into a cesspit. A wooden lavatory seat was found by archaeologists at Neatham, Hampshire, in Roman Britain.[20] This would most probably have stood over a simple cesspit. A study of latrines in use during the last years of life at Pompeii is of interest here. The author required the presence of a lavatory seat – partial or complete – as the chief criterion necessary for the

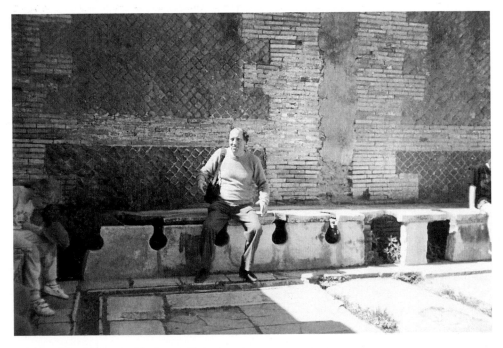

39 A marble multi-seater latrine at Ostia

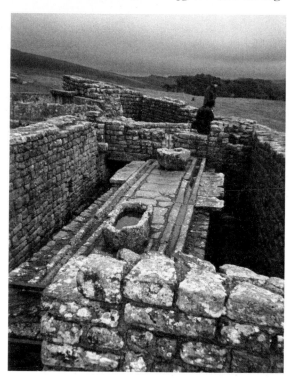

40 Latrine at Housesteads fort on
Hadrian's Wall

identification of a latrine. An additional requirement was that the room in
which the latrine was found should have a tiled and sloping floor through
which waste material could be flushed into a gully and carried away;[21] 195
latrines in various ruinous states of preservation were investigated.

The position of the latrine within the house, *domus*, was studied. More
than fifty of those examined were in or near the kitchen, a clear demonstra-
tion of the lack of understanding of even basic measures of hygiene. The risk
of food contamination in such crucially combined areas must have been high.
Other latrines were in courtyards or in the garden, or at the side entrance to
the house. Nearly all were supplied with water which could carry away the
waste matter. It was apparent to the archaeologist carrying out the research
that adequate light was an important factor, as was privacy against anyone
from outside looking in. The latter is a surprising finding in view of the many
multi-seater latrines seen throughout the Empire which could often accommodate up to sixty people on wooden or stone seats ranged around three sides
of a room. As already mentioned, such an example is to be seen at Ostia, the
ancient port of Rome. Nearer home, at Caerleon and at Housesteads (*40*) and
Chesters on Hadrian's Wall and at Bearsden on the Antonine Wall in Scotland,
similar multi-seaters are known. Nevertheless, the quantities of faecal matter
and other rubbish, which helped to preserve the Vindolanda tablets, show that
even in military establishments such conditions were less than ideal.

In the absence of lavatory paper, a sponge attached to a stick was one of the methods used for personal cleansing in the Roman world. Bowls, possibly provided for the purpose of cleaning the sponges, were found in the private latrines at Pompeii, but in most multi-seated latrines these could have been rinsed in a nearby gully through which flowed running water. If these were communal objects, as is most probable, it is easy to imagine the painful cross-infections that may have occurred, for example, in such conditions as haemorrhoids or *fistula in ano*. Such agonising conditions as these were all too common. Although seclusion seems to have been a requirement of latrines in private households, where the multi-seater public latrine is concerned this could not have been an issue. Indeed the *foricae* could have been regarded as social spaces by some, in which it may have been possible to receive invitations to dine, as illustrated in an epigram by the Roman poet, Martial.[22] A few completely intact latrines are preserved in Pompeii, but the most surprising information resulting from the research already mentioned was that latrines were found in all the different types of houses.

Research at Pompeii is continuing, in the expectation that at a further stage examination of the contents of cesspits may provide information concerning objects used or lost in the latrine, in addition to data regarding diet and diseases. Such a study, carried out at Bearsden Roman fort, on the contents of a defensive ditch, produced surprising results. The ditch had been used as a cesspit; biological and chemical analysis of the plant debris derived from faecal matter pointed to the possibility of a primarily vegetable diet. Whilst at other forts on the Wall it had been possible to excavate butchered-animal refuse pits, such pits were not found at Bearsden. No evidence for the inclusion of meat in the diet was found at the fort. However, evidence for imported food-plants, such as figs (*Ficus carica* L.), wild celery (*Apium graveolens* L.), coriander (*Corandrium sativum* L.) and opium poppy (*Papaver somniferum* L.) was seen. In addition, there were wild, edible native plants, including raspberry (*Rubus ideaeus* L.), blackberry (*Rubus fructicosus* L.), strawberry (*Fragaria vesca* L.) and bilberry (*Vaccinium myrtillus* L.). Also present were grain fragments, largely wheat. As in the Roman sewer system at York (*colour plate 18*), whipworm, roundworm and the pupae and adults of rat-tailed maggots were also present.[23]

Aqueducts, sewers and latrines were constructed throughout the Roman Empire and the towns of Roman Britain were no exception. One of the best-developed sewerage systems in any town in Britain is found at Lincoln.[24] The sewer was built in stone and roofed with stone slabs. Smaller sewers and house-drains flowed into it. At its highest point it measured 1.5m (5ft) and was 1.2m (4ft) wide. At York the sewer was no less grand.[25] It is probable that a main sewer constructed of millstone grit conducted effluent from the legionary fortress baths to the River Foss. Cleaning and maintenance could be carried out through a series of manholes which gave access to a channel 1m high and 0.45m wide. Another notable feature at York is the possible archaeological identification of a lavatory sponge in the Roman sewer.[26]

BATHS

Together with the provision of adequate drinking water and flushed latrines, a further effect to follow from the development of aqueducts in Italy and elsewhere in the Roman Empire was the adoption of baths, both public and private. These were enjoyed by Romans at all levels in society and many would have been furnished with flushed latrines where waste water from the baths was readily available to wash away the effluent. By the second century BC, many scores of aqueducts and baths had appeared throughout the Roman Empire. Numerous examples are known and have been attested by archaeological and epigraphic evidence. By the late Republican period baths had become a regular part of urban life, a habit which became strengthened during the Augustan age.[27] In Republican times people visited the baths for the purely utilitarian purpose of personal cleansing and men and women bathed at separate times. By about the time of the formation of the Principate, customs at the baths changed, as did their architecture, decoration and function. Baths became not merely places for cleansing the body, but were also stages for display, where bathers could socialise and gamble or take exercise and relax and where assignations could be made. The enjoyment of works of art was felt to be a necessary part of bathing at its best and could add to the clients' sense of well-being. This is evidenced by decorations and epigrams found in baths of all sizes.

The process of bathing included oiling oneself and scraping off the oil and dirt with a curved instrument known as a strigil. Bronze and glass *alabastra* for carrying oils, as well as strigils are found (*41, 42*). Amongst the wealthy these

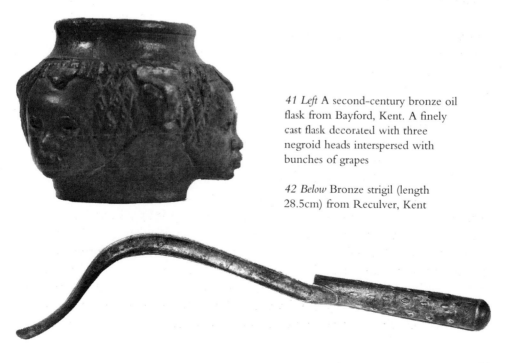

41 Left A second-century bronze oil flask from Bayford, Kent. A finely cast flask decorated with three negroid heads interspersed with bunches of grapes

42 Below Bronze strigil (length 28.5cm) from Reculver, Kent

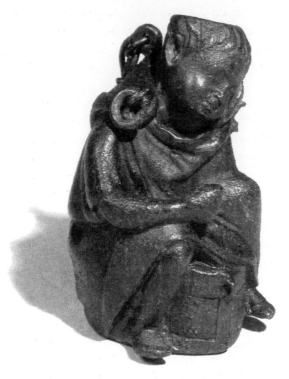

43 Bronze oil flask, from Aldborough, North Yorkshire, from the Roman town of *Isurium Brigantum*. This finely-made flask shows a young slave sitting on a box or lantern. He is perhaps waiting to accompany his master home from the baths. A small lid would have completed the head, and the remains of the looped suspension chains can be seen

would have been carried by a slave. There were beauty treatments of all kinds, as well as hair removal and massage. In addition, finds of teeth, the presence of eye stamps, catheters and other tools of the physician attest the wide variety of medical and surgical treatments that could have been available at some bathing establishments, where doctors evidently had set up shop.

Baths were not only handsomely decorated with statuary and mosaics which appealed to the aesthetic senses, but also with apotropaic symbols. These were much in demand for warding off bath demons and hostile magic and also, most especially, to avert the evil eye of envy, for naked bathers were much afraid of such negative forces. Apotropaic devices, besides being part of the baths' decor, could also take the form of personal amulets worn whilst bathing, though they were not infrequently lost, as archaeological finds attest. This is especially true of signet-rings whose stones would sometimes be lost whilst bathing, such as those found at Caerleon – in number more than eighty-eight. These are displayed in the Roman Legionary Museum, at Caerleon.

Water had its own sanctity and the religious significance of baths, and the themes with which they were decorated, also had relevance to the subject of health and medicine. This is indicated by the frequent presence of healing deities in the form of marble statuary. Although few of these marbles are extant, or have been found *in situ*, literary evidence for the presence of such deities is found in Lucian in the *Hippias*,[28] and also in the many inscriptions found in baths. Baths were adopted with enthusiasm throughout the empire and every city and town had one, or several. Baths were also provided in forts and fortresses. The activities taking place in a bath–house are described by the younger Seneca (4 BC–AD 65) whose rooms were adjacent to a bathing establishment (*Epistulae Morales* LVI.1-2, trans. R.M. Gummere).

> So picture to yourself the assortment of sounds, which are strong enough to make me hate my very powers of hearing! When your strenuous gentleman, for example, is exercising himself by flourishing leaden weights, when he is working hard, or else pretends to be working hard, I can hear him grunt; and whenever he releases his imprisoned breath, I can hear him panting in wheezy and high-pitched tones. Or perhaps I notice some lazy fellow, content with a cheap rub-down according as the hand is laid on flat or hollow. Then, perhaps, a professional comes along, shouting out the score; that is the finishing touch. Add to this the arresting of an occasional roysterer or pickpocket, the racket of the man who always likes to hear his own voice in the bathroom, or the enthusiast who plunges into the swimming-tank with unconscionable noise and splashing. Besides all those whose voices, if nothing else, are good, imagine the hair-plucker with his penetrating, shrill voice – for purposes of advertisement – continually giving it vent and never holding his tongue except when he is plucking the armpits and making his victim yell instead. Then the cake-seller with his varied cries, the sausageman, the confectioner, and all the vendors of food hawking their wares, each with his own distinctive intonation.

However, the experience not exactly enjoyed by Seneca may not have been typical of all bathing establishments. Public baths were especially important to classical medicine, especially for the Methodist sect of physicians such as Asclepiades and his pupil Themison of Tralles (*fl. c.*70 BC). In addition to helping to maintain health, baths could also alleviate the symptoms of some diseases, especially inflammations of the skin, muscles and joints.

HOSPITALS: THE ROMAN MILITARY VALETUDINARIA

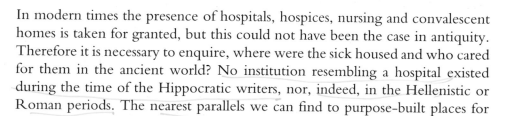

In modern times the presence of hospitals, hospices, nursing and convalescent homes is taken for granted, but this could not have been the case in antiquity. Therefore it is necessary to enquire, where were the sick housed and who cared for them in the ancient world? No institution resembling a hospital existed during the time of the Hippocratic writers, nor, indeed, in the Hellenistic or Roman periods. The nearest parallels we can find to purpose-built places for accommodating the sick are the healing sanctuaries discussed in chapters 1 and 5. However, in the Roman Empire traces of possible Roman military *valetudinaria*, or sick-bays, are found in the literary sources as well as in the archaeology of forts and fortresses.

PRIMARY SOURCES

It is especially important to observe the warnings against imposing today's establishments and practices upon those of the ancient world, when considering the subject of 'hospitals'. There is no doubt that there were places where the sick could be put up and helped; however, the problem has always been to find and to identify their actual physical remains. References to such establishments are found in primary texts amongst the writings of Cato, Caesar, Livy, Celsus, Galen, and – more specifically – Hyginus and Vegetius. Contemporary military manuals have not survived but the Roman writer Vegetius (*fl.* AD 379-95) collected the writings of ancient authorities concerning military recruitment in the Roman Army in his *Epitome of Military Matters*. This included extracts from the *De Aquis Urbis Romae* of Sextus Julius Frontinus, together with a discussion of ways in which to care for the health of the soldiers.

In addition to the source from Vegetius, the late first-century surveying manual, *Liber de Munitionibus de Castrorum*, attributed to 'pseudo-Hyginus', gives directions for selecting a suitable site on which to build a hospital. Hyginus tells us that every fortress possessed a hospital and, furthermore, that the quietest and most sheltered position within the fort or fortress should be chosen for its location. This was usually in the central range near the commanding officer's house or headquarters building, the *praetorium*. As a further means of ensuring a quiet atmosphere for the sick, wounded, or recovering soldiers, Hyginus suggests that the stables and workshop should be established some seventy Roman feet away from the hospital, 'so that it will be quiet for the convalescents'. However, based on these few sources whole edifices have been raised, for nowhere does Hyginus provide a plan for the structure and the actual physical appearance of the hospital itself remained unknown. This was the situation until an archaeologist[29] excavating a site, dated as possibly Claudian or Neronian, at Neuss (Roman *Novaesium*) between 1887 and 1901, identified a previously undetermined structure as a *valetudinarium*.[30]

ARCHAEOLOGICAL EVIDENCE

The identification of the *valetudinarium* at Neuss, on the lower Rhine, was made on the grounds that the layout of the building fitted in with plans of modern hospitals.[31] Koenen's historical identification of the *valetudinarium* at Neuss was given further impetus when, in one room of the structure, the archaeologist found a group of about a dozen medical-type instruments suspected to be probes. Moreover, even the layout of the building seemed to confirm its status. Raised hearths were discovered in what was identified as an operating theatre, where it was claimed instruments could be sterilised, and cauteries could be heated. However, although there was a general awareness of the importance of cleanliness, there could be no concept of 'sterilisation' before the discovery of the microscope and bacteriology in the seventeenth-eighteenth centuries. Hearths would have been required for heating both water and cauteries. A number of small rooms or wards, divided by hallways, were also identified. Following the identification of this building as a hospital, it was easy for other buildings with a similar design also to be designated as such, even when they did not accord with the precepts set down by Hyginus.

In addition to the archaeological findings there was environmental evidence at Neuss demonstrating the possibility that medicinal plants were cultivated in the courtyard garden at the hospital.[32] Carbonised remains of *Hyoscyamus niger* (*solanaceae*), henbane; *Hypericum perforatum*, St John's wort; *Plantago* (*Plantaginaceae*), plantain; *Centaurea* (*Compositae Asteraceae*), centaury; and *Trigonella foenum-graecum*, fenugreek, were discovered there. The potential uses of the plants are discussed elsewhere. If they were deliberately cultivated, then the idea that the structure was indeed a hospital is given further credibilty.

Several buildings identified as possible military hospitals are found on the Rhine-Danube frontiers (*44*) and others are known in Britain (*45*). All so-called legionary hospitals follow the same basic plan in which a double row of about sixty pairs of rooms, with an open corridor running between them, are ranged around a courtyard. The architecture of such buildings has been reconstructed from plans recovered at excavations where finds of medical and surgical instruments, often in conjunction with pottery and glass vessels, allow their identification as a 'hospital'. However, it is emphasised that this type of so-called 'secure' evidence is found at very few examples of such sites. Indeed, hospitals have been attested in forts in Britain and elsewhere where no such evidence was available. Examples are those at Fendoch and in the fortress at Inchtuthil. Conversely, instruments are found in other places, such as in disaster sites, burials, ritual deposits, stray finds and workshops. Thus, it has to be accepted that instruments do not necessarily indicate the presence of hospitals.

On the strength of the discoveries at Neuss, however, those who have written about hospitals[33] seem to have reached a consensus regarding the subject. A full account of these structures accompanied by details of excavation reports and aerial photographs is available.[34] All assumptions regarding buildings styled as 'hospitals' need to be challenged and the evidence rigorously re-assessed. In many cases, too, it seems that the building often designated as a 'hospital' could have served additional or alternative purposes; for example,

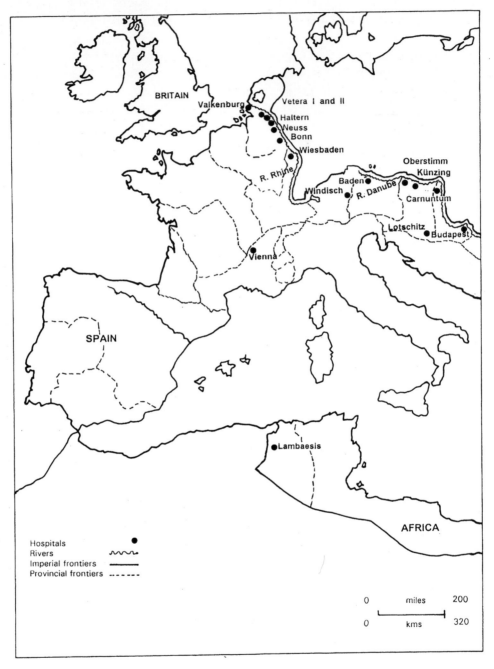

Hospitals ●
Rivers 〰〰〰
Imperial frontiers ——————
Provincial frontiers ------

| 0 | miles | 200 |
| 0 | kms | 320 |

44 Above A map showing the sites of suspected military hospitals along the Rhine and Danube. *After Majno, 1975*

45 Opposite A map showing the sites of suspected military hospitals in Britain. *After Majno, 1975*

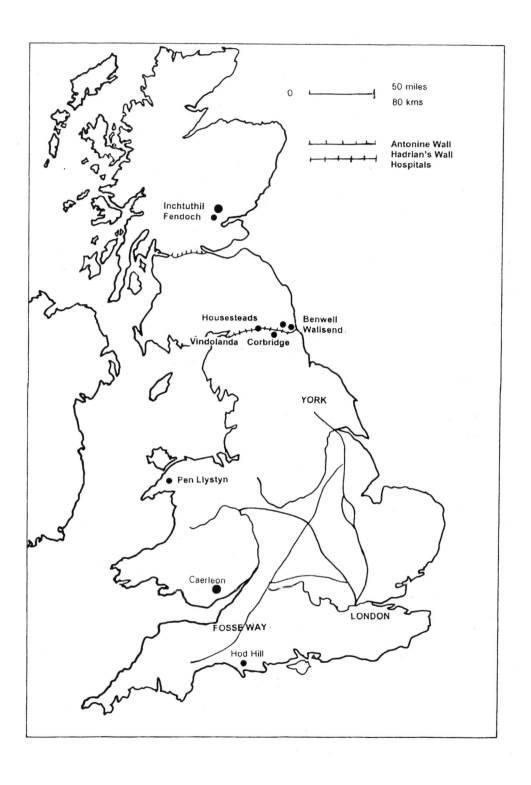

0   50 miles
                 80 kms

                 Antonine Wall
                 Hadrian's Wall
                 Hospitals

Inchtuthil
Fendoch

Housesteads   Benwell
                Wallsend
Vindolanda   Corbridge

YORK

Pen Llystyn

Caerleon

                       LONDON
FOSSE WAY

Hod Hill

the 'hospital' at *Novae*[35] on the Lower Danube in Moesia Inferior. Here, sacred statuary was found depicting the healing deities Asclepius and Hygea, as well as a small shrine dedicated to Jupiter and Minerva. This could have been a temple, or a sanctuary, or a place of healing which included a hospital.

Buildings designated as hospitals have been subjected to archaeological research at both the Augustan fortresses, *Vetera I* on the Heuneberg near Xanten (*46*), and *Vetera II Bonna* (Bonn). An Augustan structure is found at *Lauriacum* (Haltern), and at *Vindonissa* (Windisch), where a stone hospital replaced a former timber one. Other legionary hospitals are known at *Carnuntum* (Petronell) and Lotschitz in Inner Pannonia Superior, *Aquincum* (Budapest), *Vindobona* (Vienna), *Novaesium* (Neuss), and at *Novae* on the lower Danube in Moesia Inferior, the last two already mentioned above. In Britain, although excavations have been less extensive, hospitals are suspected to have been constructed at the legionary fortresses at Inchtuthil and Caerleon. Moreover, other types of evidence allow for the suspicion that hospitals could have existed at Chester and Vindolanda. Despite all the problems of interpretation, all the sites and structures mentioned above possess evidence which allows their possible identification as hospitals. Some of the most striking features of a few of these buildings will be discussed.

Finds of recognisable surgical instruments in association with these buildings suggest the status of 'hospital'. They also enable parallel buildings elsewhere to be so identified, especially where there are no such finds. However, there are some reservations, even here, since medical instruments are found in other sorts of buildings, whilst courtyard-style buildings have multiple uses. On the other hand, the single wing corridor-type construction is also the type of building used for the workshop (*fabrica*). However, on recalling the pragma-

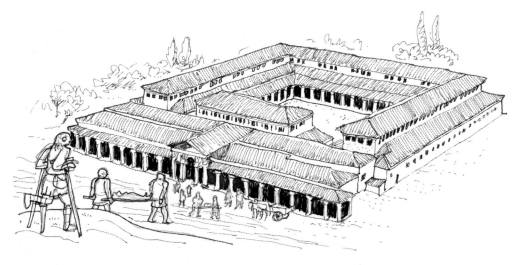

46 Drawing of the "proposed" hospital in the double legionary fortress at *Vetera* (Xanten), first century AD

tism of the Roman Army, if what the Roman military authority wanted was a storeroom, a workshop or a hospital, it is certain that such a building would have been quickly and efficiently established. Furthermore, on the subject of odd finds of surgical instruments, it is suggested that, just as in the ancient world everyone knew a little about medicine, so anyone who could afford to do so owned a few surgical instruments. This could account for some of the many stray finds. Another suggestion for these is that of ritual deposition.

Other sorts of 'hospital-type' buildings are recorded at auxiliary forts holding a *cohors* or *ala*. These were built on a smaller scale. In these smaller *castra* two types of building have been identified. The first resembles one wing of a courtyard plan. Examples are those at Oberstimm in Germany and at the wooden Agricolan fort at Fendoch, near Crieff. The second type of hospital within an auxiliary fort is a scaled-down version of the legionary courtyard model, usually found where the fort is built of stone. Possible examples of this type of building in Britain are those in the *praetentura* at Hod Hill and on Hadrian's Wall in the central ranges at Housesteads, Benwell and Wallsend. Such hospitals are also known on the *limes*, or frontier, of Germania and Raetia, and at the Valkenburg, where the fort is Claudian, built according to the courtyard plan. Similar evidence is also found at the Domitianic fort at Wiesbaden and Künzing-Quintana (late first century), built to the single-wing plan.

At *Vetera I*, present day Xanten, the fortress was designed to hold two legions (V and XXI). Built between AD 47 and 54, the hospital is the largest in the Roman Empire. It has been fully excavated and is well known in detail. The plan is in most respects typical of the courtyard-style layout suspected to have been used in legionary fortresses. In particular it bears a close resemblance to the structure at Neuss. The hospital is described as possessing colonnaded rows of rooms, a reception ward and an operating theatre. Next to this was a room where there had been hearths which could also have served a number of purposes in connection with the functioning of a hospital. A corridor ran from one side of the long hall to the other where there may have been kitchens, cooking ranges and pantries. On the west side were hot and cold baths, latrines and rooms that could have served as treatment areas. Although there were no small finds at *Vetera* to support its identification as a hospital, analysis was achieved through comparison with the structure at Neuss. The fortress at *Vetera II* also, possibly, has a *valetudinarium*. It was the replacement fortress after *Vetera I* was destroyed by Civilis in AD 70. *Vetera II* was Vespasianic but continued into the second century, at least.

The legionary fortress at Vindonissa (modern Windisch in Switzerland) has yielded a large number of surgical instruments. Although some are broken, they have mostly survived in good condition. Since the instruments were scattered throughout the fortress it is not possible to identify where medical treatment was given. A large number of instruments were found in a waterlogged deposit outside the fortress in an area called a *Schutthügel,* or rubbish–dump. Since such instruments were not intended for recycling, a ritual dimension is suspected.[36] Another site which displays unusual features is the structure identified as a *valetudinarium* at Haltern. It is dated to the late first century BC and was probably built for the campaigns of Drusus. A courtyard–style building, it was situated in the *praetentura* and oriented north–south. The lid of a box inscribed *Ex Radice Britannica* was found at the fort near the *principia* and dated to AD 14–16.[37] Not only did this cause debate about the chronology of the fort, it also pointed to the possibility of the exchange of knowledge of plants and herbal medicines between the priestly caste known as Druids, natives of Britain and Gaul (Pliny, *Nat. Hist.* 25.20–21 and 30.4.13).

INCHTUTHIL

At Inchtuthil[38] the fortress was left unfinished, although brief occupation of no more than three years, possibly by builders, is attested by finds of Samian Ware in the storeroom. The large courtyard–style hospital, similar in many details to the hospitals at *Vetera* and Neuss, was essential for possible campaigns, but in the event was not required. A probable reason for this was that troop movements in the Danube region led to soldiers being taken away from Britain. The transfer of the second *Adiutrix* to the Danube area left Chester unoccupied; *Legio XX* was therefore recalled to hold Chester. From the sequence of historical events, it was calculated that the evacuation of Inchtuthil occurred in the late summer of AD 86 or in the spring of AD 87. There were no finds of medical equipment. The timbers used in building the fort were removed, leaving only the post–holes in the ground. Archaeologically this was of great value because, despite the systematic clearance, all evidence was not lost. Modern techniques of excavation uncovered a fine example of functional architecture in the form of the post–holes. The design of the hospital may have allowed for efficient ventilation, but it would have been extremely cold and draughty. There was a central corridor with two flanking rows of small wards built as separate units. Although some scholars suggest that each corridor had a gabled roof, more recent investigations have discovered the presence of gutters and these imply that the space between the two walls was open to the sky.

Despite the difficulties of excavating the huge timber hospital at Inchtuthil, no other hospital in Britain is as fully investigated or as well described as this. Today Inchtuthil is the second largest hospital known in the Roman Empire (the largest was at *Vetera*). Its size exceeded all other buildings in the fortress. Occupying an unusually large area of 0.87 per cent of the total area. Inchtuthil had sixty–four rooms and more space could have been found if required.

The fortress at Caerleon is Flavian in date. Its 'hospital' was identified in 1964.[39] Although it was not extensively excavated, indeed the area explored was quite small, such evidence as is claimed for its existence is not supported by the structural evidence. The finds of surgical instruments were few and scattered throughout the fortress and barrack buildings. On the other hand, the building identified as a hospital at the auxiliary fort at Housesteads, on Hadrian's Wall, has been the subject of several archaeological excavations and discussions, over a period of fifty years.[40] Built in the courtyard style, it is primarily of the Hadrianic period although later modifications were carried out. In plan the structure is a smaller version of the commanding officer's house, with its rooms ranged round a central courtyard. In the absence of artefactual evidence for the practice of medicine, however, it is difficult to find reasons why this structure should not be identified as another residence. The presence of hearths, some with intense burning, perhaps suggests the possibility of kitchens. Metal-working could also have been carried out here, in which case it is possible to interpret the building as a workshop or an armoury.

Close by Hadrian's Wall, at Vindolanda, the presence of a hospital begins to emerge from the primary textual sources known as the Vindolanda tablets. These documents, preserved for almost 2,000 years in the detritus of daily life at the auxiliary fort, provide a rare and lively source of private and personal, as well as administrative, information. The military documents include important texts relating to the strength and the activities of the units stationed at Vindolanda in the period between AD 90 and 120, as well as routine reports. The thin slices of wood, on which writing in ink can be seen and read, often with some difficulty, have been excavated and interpreted by scholars over many years.[41] Some of them have relevance to the subject of medicine.

*Tab. Vindol.*156.2[42] refers to the thirty builders who had been sent 'to build a guest-house for Marcus the *medicus* (*hospitium Marco medico faciendum*). Even if he had been a 'travelling doctor', the *medicus* would at least have needed rooms while attending soldiers at the fort. In addition, it is possible to infer the presence of a hospital from the remarkable strength report (*Tab. Vindol.*154.21–5)[43] (*47*) which, as a source of information for military organisation, is perhaps the most important military document ever to be found in Roman Britain. Here information is provided that unwell soldiers, comprising over 10 per cent of those present at the fort, were separated into categories: ten men who were suffering from *lippitudo*, chronic inflammation of the eyes, were segregated from both the fifteen sick and the six wounded men. Thus thirty-one soldiers who had been removed from their quarters would have required alternative accommodation. In view of the contents of the strength report, it is no surprise to find that a hospital is referred to in another document (*Tab. Vindol.*155.6) where a reference to the *valetudinarium*, '[. . .] a [. . .] ualetudinar[. . .]' is seen.

A further writing tablet, from the archaeological context of the *praetorium*, consisted of two incomplete fragments (Inv. No.93.1350). On each of

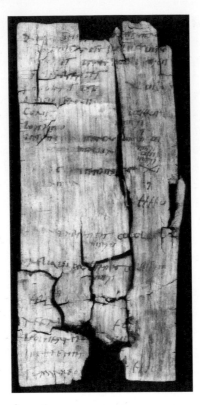

47 The strength report from Vindolanda

them was inscribed lists of substances, such as foodstuffs and minerals as well as medicaments. The documents were first considered to be inventories of basic medical supplies to be kept in the commander's residence, or perhaps in the *valetudinarium*.[44] All the substances named on the list are mentioned in the works of ancient physicians and pharmacists.[45] However, the latest theory (information from Professor Bowman) is that the fragments are now thought to be two Celsian medical prescriptions. On the first part, named 'a', the list is longer and includes more items with a known medicinal use, than those found on list 'b'. A short discussion of these now follows. 'Bull's glue' was used as a plaster for 'lichens' on the skin (possibly eczema or psoriasis); resin, too, is listed. Many plants provide this and, used with other substances, it serves the same purpose as the bull's glue. Celsus (*De Med.* V.19.1) writes of a plaster to stop bleeding which contained scraped verdigris, alum, pitch (bitumen) and scraped pine-resin. Bitumen is used for dressing wounds, or, floated on hot water, it could have been used as an inhalation to ease breathing in respiratory ailments, a hazard which may have been prevalent in that area. Chest infections would probably have been common illnesses in Britain, particularly in winter, as indicated by the importation from Italy of medicated wines, such as those found at Carpow and Caerleon. Verdigris, used in a plaster, as above, or scattered on suppurating wounds, was already an ancient remedy in early

Greek medicine. Both 'iron rust' and 'bronze rust' were known to be good for cleansing sores.

Other substances named, such as mustard seed, cumin and (on list 'b') nuts, where the skins only were used, were all ingredients which, mixed with wine, provided remedies for gastric upsets and diarrhoea. Bandages soaked in honey, also listed, could have been used to treat skin diseases such as psoriasis, ulcerating leg-wounds, varicose veins or aching joints. Moreover, the presence of honey-bandages is an indication that the list was either a prescription or an inventory, rather than an order prepared for a merchant. It would have been easier for these to have been made in the locality, perhaps in the civilian settlement, *vicus*, or in the camp, *castra*, rather than to transport them from some distance since during this time they would surely, deteriorate. Juice from oak galls, which contains 50-70 per cent tannin, was used as an astringent and a styptic; Dioscorides informs us that 'it stops the running of the gums'. On list 'b' *anesis* is interesting; it is a Greek word meaning 'the abatement of symptoms', therefore *anesi*, which is the plant fennel, was probably a 'cure-all'. According to Dioscorides, mixed with wine it was good for coughs. He also says of wheat (list 'b') 'wheatmeal has warm and drawing qualities and is nourishing'. Beans and grapes would have had their uses as foods good for recuperating convalescents. The last item on the 'b' list, potash, is an alkaline substance of vegetable origin, used in salves of all kinds.

The possibility that the lists were medical prescriptions is given further credibility, not only by the presence of the *medicus* Marcus at Vindolanda, who may well have been equipped with a clinic in addition to a hospital, either in one building or in two separate structures, but also by the find of a new tablet, to be published in *Tab. Vindol.*III, No.586.ii.pp.38, which refers to the *seplasiarius* (pharmacist) Vitalis. Another *seplasiarius*, probably peripatetic, from Carlisle (*Luguvalium*), is attested in the find of a fragment of a stylus writing tablet at Carlisle (*48*). It was found below Tullie House Museum, in silt

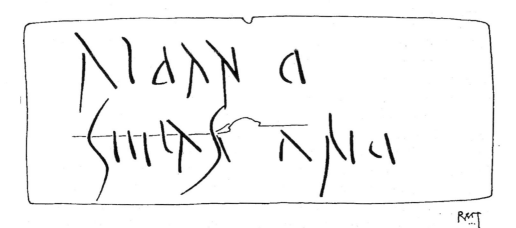

48 A fragment of a stylus writing tablet from Carlisle

filling a hollow in cobbles laid over a first-century military ditch and it reads
'*ALBAN O / SIIPLASI ARIO / [...]*' *Albano / seplasiario*, 'To Albanus the
pharmacist (?)'.[46] If Albanus was contemporary with the *medicus* Marcus, and it
cannot be assumed that this was so, he may have been a travelling pharmacist
who could have supplied Marcus the *medicus* with those ingredients named on
the prescriptions, in addition to freshly made honey bandages.

In conclusion, although it is possible at many of these sites to make a good
argument for the identification of a hospital, there is virtually no unequivocal
evidence in any of them to prove the case. However, the presence of surgical
instruments as evidence for the recognition of hospital buildings carries some
weight, even when given the caveats set out above, and likewise, of course,
with reference to the documentary evidence from Vindolanda. The much-
vaunted fitness and efficiency of the Roman Army points to health-checks for
the fit, as well as care for unwell soldiers. This is demonstrated in the strength
report from Vindolanda. Therefore, considering the archaeological, documentary and literary evidence together, it is probable that sick-bays, hospitals,
or *valetudinaria*, did indeed exist within forts and fortresses but possibly not in
every case in the situations or in the forms in which they are claimed to have
been found. However, when Roman rule ended, the military *valetudinaria*
became forgotten and the motivation to provide hospitals for the sick then
came from religion.

In the Roman world, places were set aside for sick slaves in their masters'
households, probably in a building specially made for the purpose which might
also be called a *valetudinarium*. These quarters, like the military *valetudinaria*,
existed for a particular class of person, i.e. soldiers and slaves. Hospitals for
civilians had to wait for the arrival of Christianity. Early Christians regarded
the care of the sick as their special duty. An account of Christian service, *c.*AD
150, indicates that a collection was made every Sunday 'for orphans, widows,
... the sick ... strangers'. (Justin Martyr, *First Apology*, i.67). A bishop must
be 'given to hospitality' (1 Tim. iii.2; Titus i.8), and if the bishop's house
was inadequate to accommodate his many messengers and visitors, it then
became necessary to establish a separate house for strangers, a *xenodochium*.
This, briefly, is the beginning from which the civilian hospital developed.

Although the Emperor Julian renounced Christianity and tried to revive
paganism, he continued to promote the idea of *xenodochia* in imitation of the
Christian ideal. These became familiar institutions of the Church, spreading
rapidly in the Eastern Empire. The most famous was that founded by St Basil
of Caesarea in Cappadocia, who constructed a hospital in AD 372 in which
there was rehabilitation of patients, as well as a training scheme for the staff. In
a letter Basil describes this as 'a place for the entertainment of strangers, both
for those who are on a journey and for those who require medical treatment
on account of sickness ... a means of giving these ... the comfort they want,
nurses, physicians ...'. (Basil, letter to Elias, No. xciv).[47] In the West hospitals

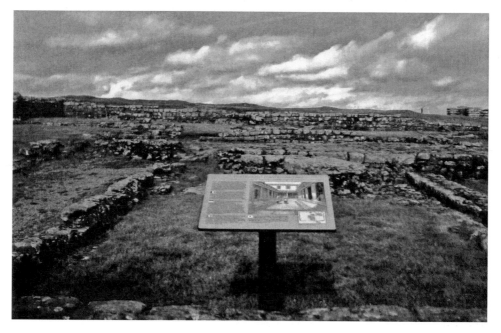

48a The Hospital at Homesteads fort. *Courtesy of David Gilbert*

spread slowly. The first infirmary was founded at Rome by Fabiola, *c.*AD 350, a wealthy widow who embraced Christianity and created a home for the sick. Thus the practice of medicine was placed in a Christian environment. This attitude of concern for the sick was a new approach. St Jerome provides the information that Fabiola went into the streets and 'carried on her shoulders wretched beings with leprous arms, swollen bellies, shrunken thighs, dropsical legs, … their flesh gnawed and rotten and squirming with little worms … How often did she wash the pus of festering wounds that others could not bear to see?'[48] In Britain, however, hospitals as such, where the sick could be cared for and fed, were unknown until the medieval period.

～5～

ROMAN DISEASES AND HEALING I
CULT

> There is a grove below the Aventine, dark with the shade of holm-
> oaks; at the sight of it you would say, 'there is a deity there'.
>
> Ovid, *Fasti* III, 295-6

Just as in the medieval period the principle behind many hospitals with a religious foundation included praying for divine aid, so in antiquity the primary aim of those attending healing sanctuaries was to achieve health through the active intervention of the gods; furthermore, in both cases, medical practitioners were probably at work. Fundamentally, therefore, the art of healing springs from a religious impulse. Although votive objects and cures sought at sanctuaries and watery places are the main focus of this chapter, according to literary sources the Roman world was beset by deadly pestilences so these, too, will be considered. The chapter also includes evidence for possible 'specialist' centres such as eye-shrines or sanctuaries which seemed to be frequented by pilgrims with injuries to the hands and feet, or others where the most prevalent anatomical votives were of the reproductive organs.

Roman populations, inevitably, inherited the epidemic diseases that had evolved during the Neolithic period, c.5000-4000 BC, when people ceased living as hunter-gatherers and led more settled lives as agriculturalists and pastoralists. These earlier peoples lived with their animals, close together under the same roof, breathing the same air and dust, touching animal waste and butchering their bodies. The dangerous inter-mix of pathogens was further encouraged by the use of animal wool and skins and the consumption of eggs, milk and flesh. Thus, new types of diseases were created. Such diseases, which pass from animals to mankind, are known as zoonoses. Intestinal worms (helminths), plague, tuberculosis, malaria, yellow fever and influenza all belong in this group.[1] The most recent plague-diseases which we are able to classify as zoonoses are, of course, HIV 1 and 2 and Creutzfeldt-Jakob disease (CJD), the human form of 'mad cow disease'. Almost every innovation to increase and improve the diet or health made by ancient (and modern) peoples, invites new infections. What is certain is that those early forms of diseases which today are identifiable were in ancient times attacking new, human, 'virgin-soil' populations – people who had no inherited resistance, no knowledge of the sources from which the diseases sprang and no means of prevention. Smallpox is now eradicated and measles and chickenpox have become the childhood illnesses familiar to us today; these are milder forms of those earlier plagues, which now give immunity to further attacks.

Unlike the great plague of Athens in the fifth century BC, which had been a contained, local infection, the Antonine Plague reached every corner of the Roman Empire during the second century AD. Whole populations were ravaged. Historically attested individuals, including emperors, died. Social and political life was destroyed. Some individuals may have ascribed the disease to bad air, or *miasma*, but public authorities continued to cast the blame for plague and famine, with all its terrifying accompanying effects, on the gods. Processions with sacrifices to city-protecting deities were staged, amulets were worn and astrology and divination were practised. Although in folk-consciousness veneration of ancient gods and goddesses was chiefly connected with the seasons, people were well aware of unknown forces that caused pestilence, injuries and accidental meetings, shaping and determining their lives. Today such events are attributed either to good fortune or to bad luck, but in ancient times they could be thought to be caused by intervening spirits, who possessed the power to safeguard, or else to cause harm to individuals and who, therefore, required propitiation.

ROMAN DEITIES

Both archaeological and literary sources attest the fact that deities and their sanctuaries flourished everywhere in the Roman world. Some deities are more ancient than the legendary foundation of Rome itself, their beginnings extending back in time beyond the reach of history. Others, such as the Greek god of medicine, Asclepius, were introduced later. Bacchus (the usual Latin title for the Greek god of wine, Dionysus (*colour plate 23*)) was present in Italy from Republican times, where he was also known as Liber and had a huge following. Ceres was a native Italian deity, representing the reproductive powers of nature. She was associated with Tellus, the earth goddess, and was especially important to agriculture and general prosperity. Romans worshipped and sacrificed to her in their fields and orchards.

Although Mars was venerated as the Italian god of war, second only to Jupiter in the Roman pantheon, he was essentially protective of (amongst other aspects of the world) wild places, lush pastures, agriculture and horse breeding.

Silvanus, god of gardening, orchards and hunting, was sometimes venerated in his own right and sometimes equated with Mars. The seasonal festival, the *lustratio*, a ceremony of purification and protection from evil influences affecting the fields, was an essential part of food production for the survival of ancient societies. The Elder Cato, in his handbook on agriculture (*De Agricultura*, LXXXIII), quotes a prayer to be addressed to Mars Silvanus by farmers at this time. The month of March, named after the god, witnessed the rebirth of the agricultural year. His altar was in the Campus Martius and a temple dedicated to Mars, *c.*390 BC, stood on the Appian Way, outside the city. Mars, as a god of fertility, was conflated with several native deities, particularly the Celtic gods of Gaul and Britain.

Cybele, the Great Asian earth-mother (*Magna Mater*) was famous throughout the ancient world, and, with her lover Attis, was known in Rome from about 204 BC. She was primarily a goddess of fertility and wild nature. She could also cause or cure diseases. Her temple was on the Palatine, but the cult, which included ritual castration, was barred to Roman citizens until the reign of Claudius. Nevertheless the worship of Cybele became part of the Roman state religion, and was also one of the most important mystery religions of the Roman Empire. The cult of Mithras was another popular mystery, flourishing especially from the second century AD, while the cults of Isis, Serapis and Harpocrates found favour with the army. In sum, the Graeco-Roman gods and imported deities from the East were ever-present saving powers to the Romans. Other gods and goddesses are much less well known but have an even greater interest in connection with healing, although some are so obscure that they are attested in only a few literary sources.

Dea Febris, goddess of fever, possessed three temples at Rome, one of which was situated on the Palatine hill, the possible site of Rome's (legendary) settlement by Romulus, testifying, perhaps, to the antiquity of the cult.[2] Carna looked after people's hearts, stomachs and general well-being. Her temple on the Caelian hill was founded in the first year of the Roman Republic, 510 BC. The Italian goddess of health was Salus, and under her name the Romans venerated several other godesses, one of whom was Fortuna. She was worshipped, for example, at Glanum in southern Gaul, where she was named Valetudo, from which the name for Roman military hospitals, *valetudinaria*, derives. Her temple on the Quirinal Hill at Rome was dedicated in the year 305 BC. Continuing archaeological excavations at Glanum are focusing on the extensive cult wells. Recent excavations have uncovered a Roman forum, a theatre and thermal baths.

Childbirth had its own protectors. These were Alemona, guardian of the foetus, and Partula, who presided over the delivery. Vagitanus secured the first, life-affirming cry of the infant and Cunina watched over the cradle. Rumina, a Dea Nutrix, safeguarded breast-feeding.[3] In private houses the Lares presided. These were gods of the farm, household and hearth, and all that belonged there. Lares were guardians of roads and crossways, too. Moreover, as told by Ovid, there were the Manes, restless spirits who, it was feared, unless appeased at their festival in February, could spread death and destruction. The presence of these gods, with their particular spheres of interest, demonstrates that people considered fevers, abortion, death of a mother during childbirth, lack of mother's milk, deaths in infancy, plague, disease and famine, loss and ill-luck in general, to be of divine or demonic origin.

Augury was a widespread practice; this depended upon readings of the heavenly bodies and the flights of birds. Haruspicy, a custom inherited from Etruria, persisted through Roman times. The *haruspex*, such as Marcius Memor, who set up a dedication to Sulis at Bath, studied the livers and entrails from sacrificial animals in order to achieve prophetic visions. It is hardly surprising, therefore, given such a degree of religiosity and dependence upon deities of all tempers, in particular those whose sphere of influence came within the ambit of procreation, agricultural success, and health and healing, that when the cult of Aesculapius was introduced to Rome from Greece in 291 BC, it was so very readily absorbed into Roman culture, ultimately becoming dispersed throughout the Empire.

HEALING SHRINES

More than 100 healing sanctuaries are known in Italy. The majority are found in the western-central areas, southern Etruria, Latium, and within the environs of Rome. Not all of them were presided over by Asclepius (*49*), for other deities, such as Diana at Nemi, assumed healing powers. Such sanctuaries would become centres for pilgrimage and many possessed appropriate accommodation where pilgrims could stay overnight or for prolonged visits during festivals. Many of the sites coincide with a layer of volcanic rocks that was abundantly supplied by mineral springs. In antiquity they served as the natural focus for healing sanctuaries and even today several of these *fontanili* are sources of bottled mineral waters.[4] Although healing deities were most often associated with water, gods and goddesses resided everywhere in the natural world. In *The Metamorphoses* Ovid tells of the close affinities which existed between human and divine spirits and the spirits of nature. Deities lived in trees, brooks and meadows as well as in caves, springs and forests and in the air.

GIFTS TO THE GODS

Shrines of healing deities are identified by finds of anatomical votives and ex-votos. The two terms are slightly confusing but it is possible to attempt an explanation. Although it is unclear whether the offer of an anatomical votive

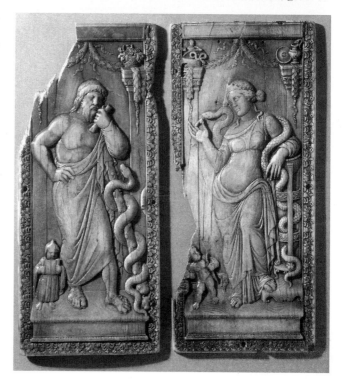

49 Asklepios and Hygea carved in Late Roman style on an ivory *diptych,* possibly serving as a portable shrine to its ultimate owner; *c.*AD 400, from Rome

represented a request for assistance, or a 'thank you' to the god for help already received, it is probable that in most cases it was the former. Whilst some anatomical votives illustrate specific pathology, the majority carry no such information. One researcher[5] felt that this was of secondary importance to the offer of the limb itself. Ex-votos, on the other hand, represented the offer of a gift to the divinity in exchange for a favour already received, which would have been either a complete healing, or merely the alleviation of symptoms.

An inscription from Piacenza, in northern Italy (*CIL*.XI.295), describing L. Callidius Primus' presentation to Minerva of two silver ears in gratitude for a successful cure, may be interpreted in several ways. It was either in payment for the cessation of ear-ache, the severe pain suffered during a middle-ear infection; or for curing a boil or something similar in the outer ear. Another possible reason for the *donatio* may have concerned the restoration of hearing. Whatever the focus of the request, the devotee would wish to express thanks to the goddess simply for listening to the prayer. On the other hand, Minerva was goddess of wisdom, as well as of crafts, and perhaps the ex-voto represented a plea for clearer understanding and an improved learning ability. The analysis of votive material, therefore, depends largely upon contemporary-minded inference, despite the presence in some cases of an apparently informative ancient inscription.

The psychological effect of hot water bubbling up out of the earth would have been one of fear and wonder at the mighty powers of the divine spirits, and a spring possessing such naturally heated waters, or beneficial minerals, would become well known. A healing shrine would then grow up in that locality. Indeed, one of the principal Roman sanctuaries of the Western Empire is found in Britain at Bath in Somerset, where both of these qualities were present, and where they continue to be enjoyed today. In Roman times the deity at Bath (*Aquae Sulis*) was Sulis-Minerva, a conflation of the indigenous Celtic deity with the Roman goddess Minerva (*50*). Also in Britain, in addition to the baths and temple complex at Bath, the site at Lydney in Gloucestershire is of great interest. Here the earth and water possess rich iron deposits. In the late Roman period a temple was erected whose plan has been compared with that of a Greek Asklepieion.[6] However, the god venerated at Lydney was the Romano-Celtic Mars Nodens.

Mineral waters would have helped to alleviate one or even several ailments, including skin diseases, nervous troubles, retention of urine, constipation, the pain of rheumatic joints and other complaints. Such illnesses as these, though not psychological in causation, would certainly have been alleviated by faith, warmth and relaxation. On receiving relief, the thankful devotee may have wished to leave a gift at the shrine. The gift itself, according to primary sources, could vary from 'first fruits,' cakes and other foods, which, of course, do not survive in the archaeological record, to models of the afflicted part of the body. These were shaped in ivory, metal, marble, stone, wood, bronze,

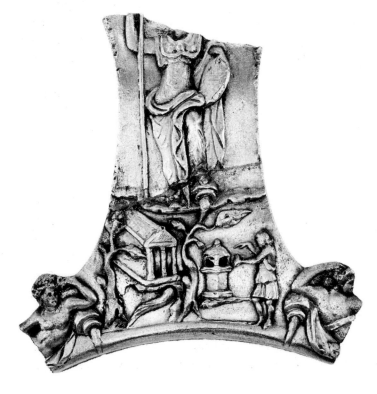

50 Silver and gilt pan handle from Capheaton, Northumberland, showing the goddess Minerva presiding over a sacred spring, possibly Bath. The source is shown symbolically issuing from a jar beneath her left foot

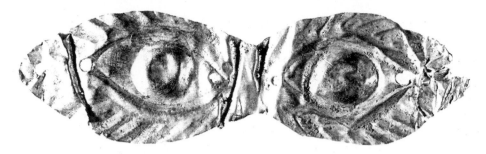

51 Gold votive eyes from Wroxeter

gold, silver or terracotta. Coins are also found and in some instances they provide dating information.

Gifts to the gods would vary in economic value, too. For example, in addition to the silver ears already discussed, there is the pair of finely-wrought gold eyes from Wroxeter, in Shropshire (found in a fourth-century AD context) (*51*). In marked contrast are the numerous, roughly-made models of eyes cut from plaster, again from Wroxeter. Furthermore, also present at this site was a collyrium stamp, indicating the possibility that a shrine once existed for the treatment of eye-complaints,[7] discussed further below. Such stamps are found at the Bath sanctuary, too, and at the Lydney temple healing complex.[8] Perhaps this was just one of several therapies that could have been available at such well-established centres of healing. Offerings in miniature are, perhaps, a consequence of scarce resources; they are, of course, symbols of the parts or items they represent. Included in this group are such items as the votive breasts made in ivory from Bath, or the scaled-down infants' feeding bottles and other pottery vessels frequently found at shrines, such as that of Diana of Nemi, or those dredged up from the River Tiber. Artificially silvered or gilded coins are present at some sanctuaries, as well as miniature weapons; in the pagan world it was accepted that the deity could turn the token object into a real one.

ANATOMICAL VOTIVES

Anatomical votives first appeared in Greece in the fourth century BC, for example at Corinth, where there was also a temple of Asclepius. First erected in the fourth century and coinciding perhaps with the adoption at Epidaurus of Asclepius, the temple at Corinth survived in different forms until late antiquity. The range of votive objects found there, made in terracotta, included all parts of the human anatomy. A fine display giving examples of many types may be seen in the small museum on the site. At about the same time, this development was paralleled in Italy, where, in addition to offerings to the major healing deities, large numbers of anatomical votives were dedicated to the minor gods and goddesses who watched over and safeguarded all aspects of everyday life. However, by the end of the Republican period (27 BC) the manufacture and dedication of anatomical votives in Italy had disappeared. Just as their arrival in the first place could have been due to the lack of an organised system of healing, their demise may have been caused, in part, by the advent of more rigorous and enquiring standards of medicine. At many of the sites, the new professional medicine already co-existed with temple-medicine.

All parts of the human body are represented (*52*). In the Etruscan area of Vulci, Tarquina, at a site known for its necropolis and for its temples and sanctuaries connected to fertility cults, more than 400 terracotta models of wombs were found (*53*). Their average size was 20cm. In many of them (around 80 per cent) the entrance to the womb was closed and in others it was open. The meaning of these differences may, perhaps, be associated with ideas connected to accidental miscarriage of the foetus, or infertility. In nearly all of the models (as may be seen on the radiograph) a small clay figure was found; in some there were two figures. These were represented by small spheres of about 1cm in diameter. The author[9] suggests that these figures are the earliest representations of intra-

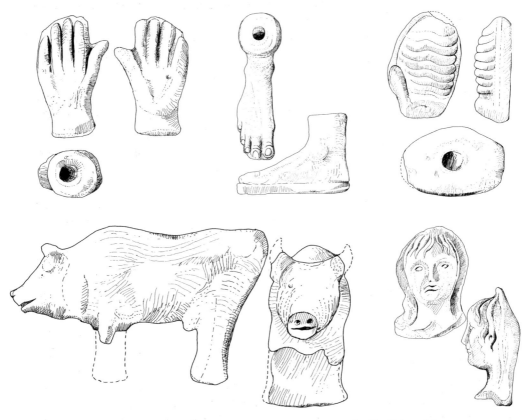

52 A group of votive objects from the sanctuary at Veii, seen in the Pitt-Rivers Museum in Oxford

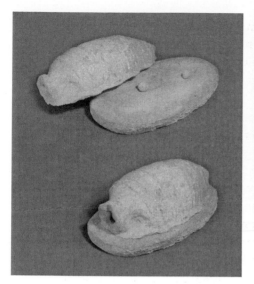 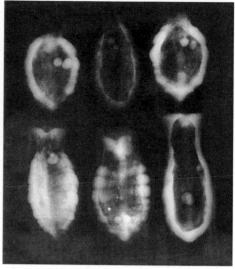

53 Votive uteri from Vulci; an X-ray shows intra-uterine figures

uterine life; they are at least five centuries earlier than the foetal positions of the *Gynaecia* of Soranus of Ephesus.

Other examples include male and female torsos, sometimes with abdominal viscera or hearts, chests, breasts, genitalia and uteri. Heads and half-heads were present at many sites complete with features, although eyes, ears, noses, tongues, teeth and hair were also presented in separate forms. In addition, there were limbs such as hands, arms, feet (*colour plate 24*), fingers and toes. Besides those votives found mainly in the western-central areas of Italy (and mostly made of terracotta) dating from the fourth to the first centuries BC, anatomical votives are known in other parts of the Roman Empire, including the Greek and Roman sanctuaries at Ephesus, Cos, Delos, Cyprus and Pergamum. At the magnificent newly constructed temple of Asclepius at Pergamum (completed *c.*AD 148) Aelius Aristides, at the request of the god, inscribed his medical experiences on written documents, a thanksgiving offering known as the *Hieroi Logoi* and a gift to the god in parallel with the inscriptions discovered at Epidaurus.

Although the practice of presenting anatomical votive objects to the gods had gone into abeyance in Italy by the end of the Republican period, it did not die out completely in the Roman world; such objects are found in the later Empire, too. Some are known in Gaul and Britain, to be further considered below. Moreover, the practice continued throughout Europe and even today the walls of Italian churches are sometimes seen to be hung with miniature ex-voto objects. In the Near East, also in modern times in Syria, at sanctuaries such as that of the Convent of the Virgin of Seidnaya, in the Byzantine town of Serjilla[10], an active healing and fertility shrine has grown up around a sacred

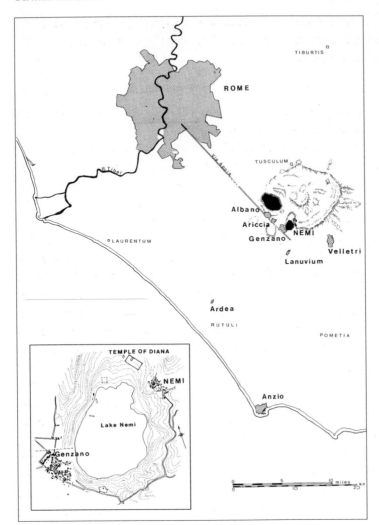

54 A plan showing
the location of the
site at Nemi

icon of the Virgin. It is supposed to have been painted by St Luke, who was a physician. Silver plaques representing parts of the bodies of pilgrims who have been healed there are also displayed. At Lourdes and at many minor springs, such as the 'virtuous well' at Trelleck in Monmouthshire, South Wales, the practice of leaving objects and clothing continues, existing today as in the ancient world, side by side with orthodox medicine.

TWO SHRINES FROM REPUBLICAN ITALY

> In the Arician vale there is a lake begirt by shady woods and hallowed by religion from of old ... no horses enter that grove. The long fence is draped with hanging threads, and many a tablet there

attests the merit of the goddess. Often does a woman, whose prayer
has been answered, carry from the City burning torches, while
garlands wreathe her brows.

                                        Ovid *Fasti* III, 266-270

One of the earliest known healing shrines in Italy is that of Diana Nemorensis
at Nemi (*54*). Archaeological evidence dates the beginnings of this shrine from
between the eighth and the sixth centuries BC. Identified by the Romans with
the Greek Artemis, Diana was goddess of woodland and fertility. As patroness
of wild beasts and nature she filled the farmers' stores with meat and fruits.
Diana the hunter-goddess wore a short chiton and boots, she carried a bow
and a clutch of arrows and was accompanied by a hound or a stag. Although
Diana is known to have occupied other sanctuaries, the one situated on the
shore of Lake Nemi at Aricia, in the Alban hills, some 26km south-east of
Rome in a sacred grove possessed of a spring, was the most famous. Geological
evidence in that locality demonstrates the frequent occurence of earthquakes
and storms, with thunder and lightning. In ancient times, the closeness of
extinct volcanoes, the woods and groves around them, as well as the possibility
of thick fog, would have given the area a spectral or mysterious atmosphere.
Lakes developed in the craters of two extinct volcanoes. They were known
as the *speculum Dianae*, the mirror of Diana. Ancient peoples developed the
belief that Rome's mystic ancestors dwelt around the woods and mountains.
Temples and shrines were set up in their honour.[11] Pilgrimages undertaken to
the site would have been extremely arduous.

Votive objects from Nemi[12] consisted largely of statuettes of single figures as
well as couples, some carrying an infant, others in which the female seems to
be pregnant. These would have been dedicated, perhaps, by devotees anxious
for fertility, or by a woman concerned for the safe delivery of a child. There
were also models of heads and half-heads, pairs of eyes, uteri, phalli, breasts
and hands and feet, all offered by people seeking cures for particular maladies.
Such objects demonstrate that, at Nemi, Diana was especially worshipped as
goddess of fecundity, childbirth and healing. They indicate that Diana not only
bestowed offspring on couples, but that she also heard the prayers of mothers
in travail. Large numbers of votives were found huddled together in pits, a
device possibly designed to retain or 'recharge' in them the power of the deity.

Archaeological excavation uncovered a late fourth-century BC temple
which was rebuilt in the second century BC, when a theatre was added. In
the first and second centuries AD, further structures of the type normally
associated with healing sanctuaries, such as baths and a theatre, were built on
the site. In the Imperial period, despite or perhaps because of, the difficulty of
access, a more fashionable and wealthy clientele was attracted to Nemi. They
included emperors and their courts. Villas and other amenities were built along
the Via Appia. Ancient literary sources[13] attest an 'almost immemorial divine

presence at Nemi'.[14] It was one of the most popular shrines in central Italy. The power and importance of the site is demonstrated by its longevity; epigraphic evidence continues into the Antonine period, whilst coins found at the site are dated as late as the fourth century AD.[15]

On 13 August, Diana's feast day, she was honoured throughout Italy. There were torchlight processions and harvest festivals, whilst at Rome great torchlit columns of women would process from the city to the *nemus* (grove). At such times 'the lakes shone with the reflections of the lights'.[16] Pilgrims from Latin communities other than that of Aricia had always been attracted to the wood at Nemi. Furthermore, Diana[17, 18] was worshipped at several other woodland groves, for example at Mount Tifata near Etruscan Capena, north of Rome. Every *lucus* was consecrated to her.[19] On the Aventine in Rome a temple was erected in her name, *c*.550 BC, where she was represented by an image of the many-breasted Ephesian Artemis, 'with all its crowded emblems of exuberant fecundity'[20] and also, perhaps, as a highly emphasised type of mother goddess (*55*). At this shrine Diana was worshipped as goddess of the moon and light – further aspects of the female principle. A place of asylum, demonstrating a nurturing function, was established in the Aventine temple. It had originally been regarded as neutral ground for the reconciliation of disputes between the Latin towns. Such rights may have been inspired by the Artemision at Ephesus; in Rome they were enjoyed by many, including fugitive slaves.[21]

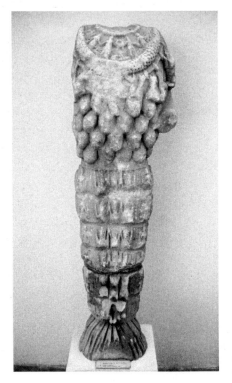

55 Statue of Ephesian Artemis from Cos

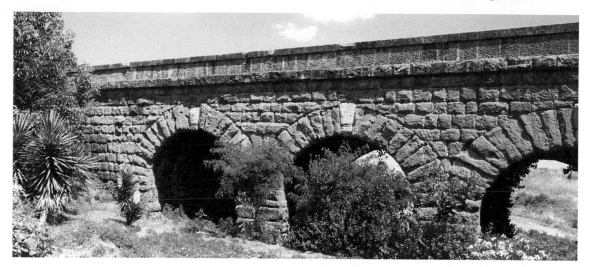

56 Part of the Republican bridge at Ponte di Nona

THE SANCTUARY AT PONTE DI NONA

Healing shrines are sometimes discovered by workmen while carrying out road or building works and some become the subject of archaeological investigation. However, in contrast to the shrines of Diana, the identity of the deity at such sanctuaries is not always apparent. The wayside shrine at Ponte di Nona is just such a case. Excavations in 1975 and 1976 yielded totals of more than 8,000 terracotta ex-votos, the majority representing whole bodies, or separate organs and limbs. Moreover, pertinent to the subject of healing, further finds included vessels whose purpose was to contain ointments, *unguentaria*.[22]

Situated on the Via Praenestina, 9 miles east of Rome, slight remains of the magnificent Republican bridge continue to be visible down to the present time. Nowadays this is heavily supplemented by modern restoration (*56*). Following preliminary excavations in 1975, in 1976 more extensive trenches were dug. These demonstrated that the site (*57*) was first occupied in the fourth century BC when brushland was cleared to make way for the sanctuary area. By the time of the second century BC, the locality had gained the reputation that it was a place of some importance, doubtless because of the magnesium-bearing spring that existed there. The shrine which grew up was known locally as *Ad Nonum*, a reference to its distance of 9 miles from Rome. From the third century AD onwards, a shrinking number of finds suggests a diminishing population. Many such sanctuaries were victims of the disruptions of late Imperial times and Ponte di Nona seems to have been one of them. Although some activity continued into the fifth century AD or later, attested by a layer of African Red-slip Ware, there was complete desertion in the early Middle Ages.

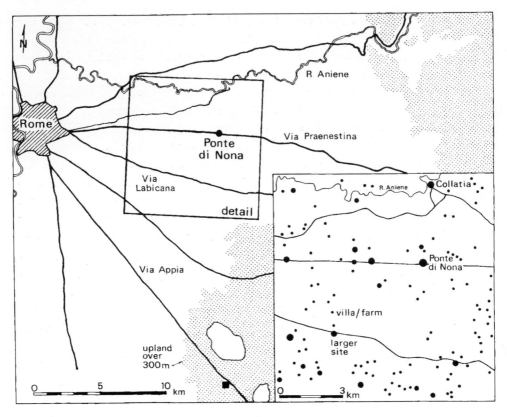

57 A map showing the location of the site at Ponte di Nona

The healing sanctuary, which had once included a temple complex, grew up on the crest of a ridge. Large quantities of terracotta anatomical votives (*c.*8,400) in addition to more than 1,500 sherds of contemporaneous pottery, including various black-glaze fabrics and a percentage of tableware, indicated the unusual nature of the deposit. It was suspected that some of it would have been used in temple ritual. Many of the terracottas were found in specially dug pits, similar to those at Nemi. Others were spread over ditches, or packed around the footings of buildings. All these discoveries point to the use of the site as a healing sanctuary and a place of pilgrimage. An enclosure measuring some 175m by 40m was assumed to be a *temenos* area, although by this time (1975/6) there was no evidence of a temple. Nearby, as at Nemi, were other types of buildings of the sort normally associated with healing sanctuaries, such as a suite of baths and several small rooms. A circular structure, 10m in diameter, made in *opus quadratum*, was interpreted as a possible pool. A cave-like nymphaeum found in this area to the east of a stream was thought to have been an outlet for the magnesium-bearing *fontanili*. The popularity and expansion of the sanctuary is attributed to its opportune position at the crossing of a route to another shrine of great importance, the enormous terraced sanctuary of the goddess *Fortuna*

Primigenia at Praeneste (modern Palestrina). An oracular shrine, the deity here was connected to fertility and good fortune.

In modern times the site at Ponti di Nona was completely destroyed. Tractor-ploughing in the 1920s was followed in 1963-4 by the excavation of a huge quarry for *pozzolano* (a type of cement) causing obliteration of the whole temple-complex and many of the surrounding buildings. However, at this point vital information was gathered and saved by Italian archaeologists, and as a result of this and later archaeological research, a major paper concerning the sanctuary was published, with an appendix in which the anatomical votives from the 1975 excavation were discussed, with particular attention to their medical relevance. The theme of the paper was stated: 'that the votive deposits... should be considered not only in terms of their art-historical interest, but also as an indication of the more prevalent ailments that afflicted the patrons of such sanctuaries'. An overview of these votives demonstrates that there are distinct groupings, implying a degree of specialisation.

It is interesting to speculate about how and where the votives were manufactured. Many of them were life-size in scale, and there were large quantities of them; these facts indicate, perhaps, the great numbers of pilgrims who attended, or passed through the shrine. They would not have been easy to transport, and were, possibly, manufactured not far from the sanctuary. It is probable that several manufactories grew up as family businesses along the pilgrim routes throughout western-central Italy. This would account for the differences in workmanship and materials. Some of the clays used were coarse, others were extremely fine; a gritty buff fabric is also found. All votives were made from moulds, some of which were worn, giving imperfect results. Other models were hastily made and of poor artistic merit. Attempts at anatomical realism were shown by the surviving traces of paint. No disease or malady of any sort was depicted on the votives at Ponte di Nona.

Some of the heads were detailed and may have been specially commissioned portraits, as such they would have been expensive. This can also be said of several of the models of feet, a few of which were so well made and life-like that they could have represented the feet of specific individuals, suggesting that the shrine was attended by different economic groups. It is probable that pilgrims came from some distance, especially if they were visiting *Ad Nonum* on their way to the shrine at Praeneste. At the time of the site's peak activity, it is possible that there may have been shops and stalls around the sanctuary also. (Such a situation was envisaged for several of the Greek shrines described in chapter 1.) Although the terracotta votives from *Ad Nonum* consisted largely of hands and feet, generally interpreted as indicating a cult that was mainly patronised by agricultural workers, other anatomical models were also present, including large quantities of eyes, as a consequence of which a centre for the treatment of eye disorders is also suspected (*58*).

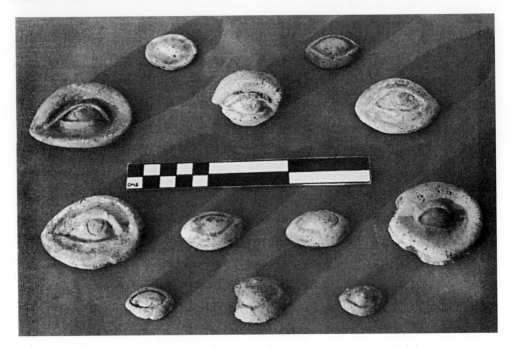

58 Votive eyes from Ponte di Nona

A MEDICAL INTERPRETATION OF THE VOTIVE TERRACOTTAS

The terracottas from Ponte di Nona are particularly interesting because they differ from those of other sites, including the mainly fertility-related models at Nemi and those from other sites disscussed below. If the nature of the disease or ailment could be known for which each ex-voto was given, this would inform us about the quality of health and the attitudes of ancient populations. In the absence of epigraphic evidence, however, a reliable interpretation is not forthcoming and we must depend on inference. The following deductions are made by an informed medical and archaeological opinion, that of the late Dr Calvin Wells. They concern only those votives discovered in the 1975 excavation.

First, there is a striking difference between the numbers of feet (752) and hands (142). Wells puts forward the theory that although in a farming community the hand is more vulnerable to injury, it is also able to heal quite easily. This would have been particularly applicable in the days before power-driven machinery, which today is often responsible for many injuries. The hand has a great capacity for recovery, too; its function can restore itself, and whilst it does so the mouth or teeth may serve as a third hand. But the feet of people in such a community are different. Ingrowing toe-nails, *hallux valgus* (bunion), and loss of the plantar arch (flat-foot), with the tender callosities and strained ligaments that accompany such conditions, are painful, and never heal spontaneously. These problems are often bilateral and although some of the votives may be accounted for by the odd clubfoot, which is usually on its own, it seems probable that feet were donated in pairs, thus accounting for the large numbers of them. We can only guess about the amount of walking required to reach the site on the part of some of these devotees; this would be a measure of the extent of their needs. It is also probable that a significant proportion of the people visiting the shrine suffered from osteoarthritis of the hands, feet, spine and hip joints; such disabilities would not necessarily be apparent in the ex-votos. Moreover, osteoarthritis is common in all communities, then as now; its relevance to ancient populations is discussed in another chapter.

The treatment of eye disease is inferred from the high number of votive eyes found at the site; in 1975 these numbered 79. Dr Wells considered that those showing the eyeball only reflected conditions affecting vision, such as myopia (short-sightedness) detached retina and cataract or squint. On the other hand, those representing eyelids and other periocular tissues could indicate infected lesions, such as blepharitis, styes, trachoma, or chronic conditions of the conjunctiva. All of these diseases are widespread in circumstances of poor hygiene and often lead to visual defects, or even blindness. Fly-borne gogno-coccal opthalmitis causes blindness in children of all ages; it spreads rapidly in any community, most particularly among children, but it also affects adults. The causal organism is highly contagious and the eyes of new-born babies are easily infected during the birth process.

Votive male genitalia from the 1975 excavation at Ponte di Nona numbered 37. However, this is a small number when compared to other anatomical parts offered at the shrine. In this situation the possibility that such votives may be present in an apotropaic sense is unlikely. Alternatively, as at other sites, there may be a connection with fertility. Much more probable, however, is an association with sexually transmitted infection, such as gono-coccal disease. The main symptoms of any venereal disease include the painful conditions of cystitis and urethritis, but other infections also cause these signs. In the healing sanctuary at Campetti in the town of Veii, in Campania, the terracottas are also associated with male and female genitalia. In addition there are breasts and a small number of hand and foot votives.[23] Again, it is possible to infer a centre where people sought either divine help for fertility problems, or cures for diseases. Moreover, in contrast to the localities at *Ad Nonum* and Paestum, Veii 'had air around it that was pure and good for people's health',[24] therefore the shrine would have been known as an especially good place to be. In such a salubrious area the illnesses of the local population would have been different, too; for at the very least, they would probably not have been subject to the symptoms of malaria, one of which is a blinding, migrainous headache.

Migrainous headaches also cause eye symptoms. A typical feature of the headache in migraine is that it affects one side of the head only. Another is the occurrence of kaleidoscopic visual disturbances known as 'castellation figures'.

These can be of blinding brilliance and intensity. Therefore, migraine could quite easily be the reason for the donations of heads and half-heads, discovered on the site at Ponte di Nona and also seen at Nemi. This theory is applicable in particular to the half-heads. As already implied above, one cause of such severe headaches is malaria, especially the cerebral type of the disease. Therefore, given the geographical location of Ponte di Nona, it is probable that some of the votive offerings were associated with malarial infections.[25]

The skin is the most vulnerable organ of the body. When it is unbroken it is a magical symbol of wholeness, a sacred gift from the gods. For the Hippocratic writers, healthy skin was the sign of a well-ordered body, conversely, unhealthy skin signalled psychological or physical disorder. Skin disease in antiquity was often seen as moral and religious pollution which it was possible to wash away through purification.[26] This outlook of fear could have been influenced by those early forms of plague-diseases and the skin eruptions to which they gave rise. It is probable that donations of limbs may have come from such people. Therefore, unsightly skin diseases, besides being distressing and irritating, are painful at many levels of experience. Besides the skin lesions of plague, a few more examples of diseases which can cause skin eruptions are eczema, scabies and fungal infections. Furthermore, finds of *unguentaria* support the suggestion that skin disease may have been a reality at *Ad Nonum*; the spring at the site possessed magnesium salts which would have been an effective treatment for many of these complaints. Indeed, in modern medical practice magnesium sulphate paste continues to be used for such disorders.

Another healing shrine was found at Paestum in Campania. Originally the Greek colony of Poseidonia, Paestum flourished in the sixth and fifth centuries BC. The Doric temples for which the city is famous were built at this time (*colour plate 25*). However, due to the flooding of adjacent marshes by a neighbouring river, as reported by Strabo,[27] Paestum became malarious. Control of the flooding streams proved all too difficult, even for the Roman public servants who were usually adept in such matters. Social customs collapsed and people began to emigrate. In the fifth century AD the Temple of Athena, which stood on the highest point of the land, was converted into a Christian church. The site was eventually abandoned in the ninth century. Rediscovered by archaeologists in the eighteenth century, votives were recovered from pits which had been continually reused in antiquity. However, although the stratigraphic sequence was thus spoiled, it was possible to date the models by style and typology. Terracotta figures such as seated goddesses and votive wombs, included types from Corinth and Rhodes, many emphasising the mysteries of sexuality and reproduction.[28]

However, at about the time of the arrival of the Romans, *c.*273 BC, new types of votives appeared.[29] Roman Juno, conflated with the Greek goddess Hera, remained the main focus of worship. Offerings included terracotta infants in swaddling clothes, apparently pregnant women and also women with newly born infants. There were numerous anatomical votives including eyes, feet, uteri and phalli, all reminders of a cult devoted to health and healing, nourishment and fertility. In the north of Paestum, Athena had been the chief deity. Her Italic name, through Roman times, was Minerva. Therefore, there may have been a cult of Minerva-Medica at Paestum. All over Roman Italy many such sanctuaries existed; a few have been discussed above and an attempt has been made to infer and to analyse the part they played in the lives of the people in the communities that they served. However, ultimately, much of this must remain conjectural.

ASCLEPIUS TRAVELS TO PLAGUE–STRICKEN ROME

Although many accidents and diseases suffered in antiquity were the same as those of today, plague was an all-pervading horror, and would have been much dreaded. In modern times, avoidance of contamination is well understood, but this was not the case in antiquity. Many of the early types of pestilence have been eradicted; new plagues, nevertheless, arise. As their effects on the course of history, on the lives of individuals and on whole populations and continents unfold before us (for example the AIDS pandemic) – even in the face of highly-developed scientific research – it becomes easier to understand the fear and helplessness of ancient peoples when confronting their own plagues. In place of 'science' they had gods, the kindliest of whom was Asclepius. The plagues which struck the Roman Empire during the third and second centuries BC, and again from the first to the fifth centuries AD, were especially devastating. Plague could have been the cause, as in 430 BC at Athens, of the abandonment of the old gods. It could also have encouraged in Rome the adoption of new gods, as described below. Eventually plague, which had brought about the end of Athenian imperialism, also contributed to the disruption of the Roman Empire; but this is to anticipate the historical and epidemiological events of which such pestilences are but a part.

When Rome was held in the grip of a plague in 293 BC, it was decided by the Roman Senate to consult the Sibylline Books. At such a time of disaster to the state, it was felt that a new god was required and the advice obtained from the writings of the oracle was to send to Epidaurus for Asclepius. The arrival in Rome of the paramount healing deity of the Greek world occurred in 291 BC. It is recorded by several authors, one of whom was the poet Ovid (43 BC–AD 17), who referred to the event in two poems. Another source, dating to the first century AD, quoted below, is in the medical papyrus known as the 'Anonymus Londinensis', now in the British Library. This document contains material ultimately derived from a medical history written by Aristotle's pupil, Meno.

The Romans, on account of a great pestilence, at the instructions of the Sibylline books, sent ten envoys under the leadership of Quentus Ogulnius to bring Asclepius from Epidaurus. When they had arrived there and were marvelling at the huge statue of the god, a serpent glided from the temple, an object of veneration rather than horror, and to the astonishment of all made its way through the midst of the city to the Roman ship, and curled itself up in the tent of Ogulnius. The envoys sailed to Antium, carrying the god, where through the rough sea the serpent made its way to a nearby temple of Apollo, and after a few days returned to the ship. And when the ship was sailing up the Tiber, the serpent leaped onto the nearby island, where a temple was established to him. The pestilence subsided with astonishing speed.[30]

The god's arrival on the Tiber island in the third century BC was a significant event for Roman medicine and also for religion. It is the first example of a foreign cult being imported directly into the Roman Pantheon; other foreign deities had been introduced via the cults of the Latin and Greek cities of Italy. Thereafter the cult of Asclepius (now Romanised and called Aesculapius) became known throughout the Roman Empire. The movement was assisted by the religious activities of the army.

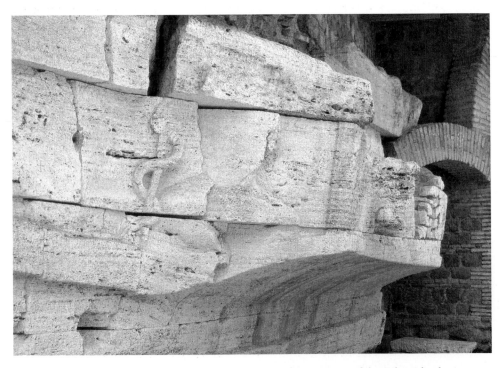

59 The relief fragment of Aesculapius on the ancient wall at the bow of the Tiber island

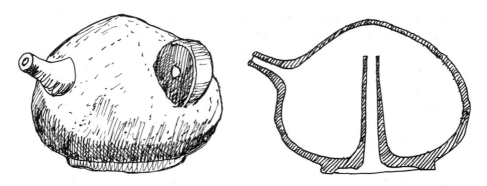

60 A Roman infant's feeding bottle from the Tiber

The Tiber island at Rome, *Insula Tiburina*, possessed of a healing spring, was already a sacred space when a temple, built in the form of a ship and dedicated to Jupiter and Aesculapius, was built there (*59*). It was restored at intervals over the centuries and was used as a depot for abandoned, elderly and sick slaves. It is not known whether care of any sort was given, although early in his reign Claudius passed a law stating that any slave who recovered whilst staying on the island would be made free.[31] It is sometimes suggested that this was an early type of hospital dedicated to Aesculapius, and there may be truth in this.[32] Later, a Christian hospital named after St Bartholomew was built on the site. This was to be influential in the medical history of the Middle Ages. It was the precursor to the great London hospital of that name, founded in the twelfth century by the monk Rahere on his return from a pilgrimage to Rome.[33] The background to the foundation and sanctity of the Tiber island is rooted in legends which have their beginnings at the time when the Etruscans ruled Rome and its subsequent history provides a notable example of the continuity of sacred space.

Following the arrival of Aesculapius at Rome, the plague subsided and, at about the same time, resistance to Greek medicine gradually became moderated. Between 1881 and 1890 the River Tiber was drained and its banks re-aligned. Huge quantities of anatomical votives were recovered, testifying to beliefs in a range of different deities. The votives came particularly from the river-bed around the area of the Tiber island. Many would have come from the site of the first temple of Aesculapius in Rome, others were of earlier date. Unfortunately for archaeology and medical history, and as in the case of the votives from Nemi, the material became dispersed when sold to local antiquaries and private collectors in Europe and America. However, a medical doctor, Luigi Sambon, acquired a few of the objects, details of which he subsequently published.[34] Many anatomical votives are described in his paper; other types, too, are discussed, such as the wedded couples with or without infants, and an infant's feeding cup (*60*). All of them are common finds at shrines

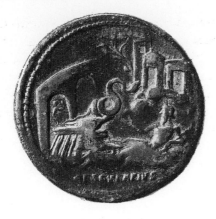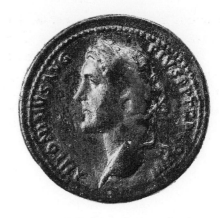

61 Bronze medallion of Antoninus Pius showing the arrival of Aesculapius at Rome

throughout Italy. The tradition of watery deposition, such as rivers and lakes, was valued as highly as that at other sorts of sanctuaries.

The adoption of Aesculapius by Rome is attested in sources other than ancient literature. During the reign of Antoninus Pius (AD 138-161), *c.*AD 143,[35] a large and handsome medallion was struck in bronze. On the obverse the head of the Emperor is portrayed and on the reverse is the River god, Tiber, reclining in the water, his right hand raised to welcome a boat passing under one of the arches of a double-arched bridge. The coiled serpent of Aesculapius sits on the prow and a human figure stands at the stern. Depicted on the island, in the background, is a tree; walls and gates are also shown. This is an impressive illustration of the arrival of Aesculapius at Rome (*61*). Other medallions depicting the god's arrival in Rome are known. The event was celebrated in literature and, later, in art and was also of great importance for religion.

The epidemic in 293 BC was neither the first nor the last of its kind to hit Rome. The historian Livy (59 BC-AD 17) recorded many such plagues during the Republican period. Thirty thousand people are reported to have died during an epidemic in AD 65, and a further plague, which struck Rome in AD 189, is reported to have caused the deaths of 2,000 people daily.[36] But it was the Antonine Plague which seems to have hammered the Roman Empire the hardest. It rampaged from AD 165 for more than fifteen years, breaking out and starting up again in different areas. Sources of the pestilence may have been infected troops returning from campaigns in the Near East, marauding tribes, too, could have been carriers, or the plague may have been spread by the activities of trade, for Rome was a maritime nation. From the second century trading routes extended to India, and in the fourth and fifth centuries as far as the steppes leading to Mongolia and China. The marauding Huns, nomadic invaders from central Asia, driving before them Vandals and Goths, poured into Italy, Spain, France and North Africa, carrying and mixing infections not met with before by some of the populations whom they over-ran. European and Asian pathogens could now meet through three new links, ships, caravans, and the Huns. Ships carried infected men, rodents, insects, and cargo. Trade along the Silk Road carried diseases both east and west.[37] The Justinian plague (to be discussed below) in the sixth century has been attributed to the ivory trade from the Horn of Africa, or rather to rats travelling with the ivory merchants to the Mediterranean.

THE ANTONINE PLAGUE

Galen and other medical writers blamed the plague on 'seeds of disease', a theory reminiscent of the teachings of Anaxagoras, in which minute 'seeds', both positive and negative ones, circulated freely in the atmosphere, and on becoming conjoined could cause putrefaction.[38] Writing in *c*.AD 189, the historian Dio Cassius (AD *c*.150-235) noted 2,000 deaths a day in Rome. Paulus Orosius (a Spanish writer, *fl.* early fifth century AD) reported complete depopulation of many towns and villages during the early years of the plague. Ammianus Marcellinus, too, described 'pollution, contagion and death'. These accounts, written, in some cases, several centuries after the events they attempt to describe, need to be used with caution.[39] During the epidemic, in AD 166, the Greek physician Galen (*c*.AD 129-216?) left Rome to return to his home in Asia Minor. Summoned to return to Rome the following year, he described the disease in his treatise *Methodus Medendi*. Galen's references were brief, his descriptions helpful neither to healers of the day, nor to modern historians. Razes, the great Persian physician (AD 865-925), on reading Galen's account, was certain that he recognised smallpox, which he knew well. However, Galen had recorded nothing about contagion, or pock-marked survivors. Nevertheless this plague became known as the 'Plague of Galen'. Scholars continue in their attempts to identify ancient diseases in modern terms and historians argue about whether plagues were smallpox, measles, malaria or typhus, or even isolated instances of bubonic plague. However, what is of greater interest is the effect of plagues on individuals and on society and any progress that may have been made in the treatment of the disease.

Nine years after the plague was thought to have ended, it broke out again. The Emperor Lucius Verus (*fl.* 161-169) died in the plague and Marcus Aurelius (*fl.*161-80), much of whose reign had been spent in the long dark shadow of it, ruled alone until his own death. Like Galen, he was away from Rome, but for a much longer period of time, commanding his legions near the Danube, where he was to write his *Meditations* before he, too, succumbed to the disease. His only reference to it is Bk IX.2, where he writes to the effect that, 'even the pestilence... is less deadly than falsehood, evil behaviour, and lack of true understanding among men'. The Antonine plague, bad as it was, turned out to be neither Rome's worst, nor its last plague. From the second century and through to the fifth, famine, migration, war and pestilence were continuous, death, devastation and desolation followed in dismal rotation. Plague and famine wiped out whole populations, the land became neglected and estates were abandoned. It is no surprise to find that the bones of peasant farmers in the late Empire show anaemia and stress fractures, all signs of poor nutrition and overwork. There could hardly have been a more powerful imperative for the cries and prayers of the people, to call out upon the gods of health, healing, fertility and agriculture.

GAUL AND BRITAIN

Evidence for the veneration of deities of healing, health and fertility and for the location of their shrines in Gaul and Britain comes largely from inscriptions. The remains of buildings, and finds of artefacts usually associated with healing sanctuaries, are also known. For example, finds of anatomical votives (unlike those made from terracotta in Greece or Italy) in these north-western provinces, are mainly made of metal or stone; wooden ex-votos are also known. As in Greece and elsewhere, such shrines are associated with watery places. Many, but by no means all, have links with the Roman Army.

Although in Italy the practice of dedicating anatomical ex-votos declined towards the end of the Republican period, the custom survived in the provinces, especially in Gaul and Britain. Sanctuaries include those at Bath, Lydney, Nettleton Scrub and probably Coventina's Well at Carrawburgh on Hadrian's Wall. A shrine also appears to have been connected with eye-complaints on the site of the Wroxeter Baths-Basilica.[40] Woodeaton and Uley, although not primarily healing shrines, are associated with healing by finds of votives; Woodeaton has a small foot and at Uley, the shrine of Mercury, the god of travellers, votive legs are found. The temple at Buxton (probably of *Aquae Arnemetiae*) has not been excavated but the name of the goddess, *Arnomecta*, is known from an altar[41] probably commemorated in the name of the Roman spa-town (*62*). In most instances the shrine would have had Celtic origins and would have been expanded later in the Roman period.

As already mentioned, at Wroxeter the presence of a shrine especially for eye diseases was suspected when a pair of gold eyes was found[43] as well as more than 35 representations of eyes cut from wallplaster.[44] The plaster eyes varied in their quality of workmanship and perhaps were made by partially sighted or blind people. Barker writes that the backs were hollowed out so that they fitted into the palm of the hand. Alternatively this shape could indicate the eye-socket. Two small temples north of the forum on the other side of West Street from the baths are known from aerial photographs and it seems that it is from here that the votive eyes may have originated. Nettleton, on the other

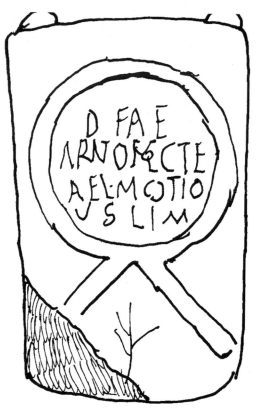

62 An altar to the goddess
Arnomecta, commemorating
the name of Buxton, found at
Brough-on-Noe in Derbyshire
(*RIB* 281)

hand, was a rural shrine dedicated to Apollo Cunomaglos, 'Hound-Prince'. It was possibly a minor spa and was in use from the early second century until about AD 330.[45] A building interpreted as a sleep-house was found, but there were no anatomical votives. The presence of an adjoining long house and the hound epithet of Apollo are reminiscent of the site at Lydney with its votive hounds and its own *abaton*, to be discussed below.

Mother goddesses also are attested in Roman Britain. There are two types, both possessing protective and nurturing functions, hence their popularity with soldiers. *Matres* occur both on inscriptions and in sculpture and are common in the Cotswolds, in Bath, and the area around Hadrian's Wall. They take various forms, often being found in threesomes and occasionally as single figures. In London a group of four has been found. These are depicted with baskets of fruit, loaves or fishes. Others are shown with nursing infants and in this case they are regarded as *Deae Nutrices*. Amongst Gallic examples is an altar depicting three buxom mother-goddesses at Lyons, dedicated by a Greek doctor Phlegon.[46] *Deae Nutrices* in pipe-clay, usually seated in a high-backed wicker chair, nursing one or two infants, were often mass-produced in central Gaul and the Rhineland and exported within the Romanised lands of the Celts, as objects of personal devotion and domestic fertility[47] (*colour plate 26*).

The infant's feeding bottle, fashioned in the shape of a female breast, found at Carlisle[48] is also of interest, for it demonstrates care for a child whom it may not have been possible to nourish by natural means. It is not dissimilar to that found in the Tiber (*60*). Without such essential human intervention, bodily health and even life itself would not be possible.

In Britain, inscriptions to deities of healing are mainly dedications to Aesculapius. A dedication (*RIB* 1052) from Publius Viboleius Secondus is found at South Shields (*Arbeia*) (not shown). Another dedication (*RIB* 1072) (*63*, bottom), this time an altar, was set up at Lanchester by the tribune, Titus Flavius Titianus; he would appear to have been literate in both Greek and Latin. *RIB* 609 (*63*, top left), by Julius Saturninus, is a dedication 'To the holy god Aesculapius and to Hygiaea, for the welfare of himself and his own'. It is a rare example in which the goddess of health appears in Britain under her

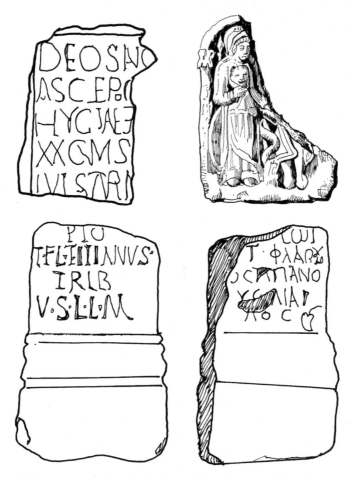

63 Some inscriptions from Roman Britain showing dedications to healing deities. Top left, *RIB* 609; top right, *CSIR* 85; bottom left *RIB* 1072 (front); bottom right *RIB* 1072 (reverse)

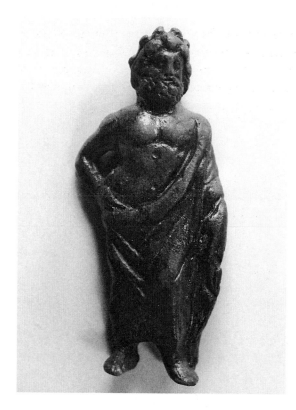

64 A small bronze figurine of
Aesculapius from Sussex

Greek name. A dedication to Minerva and Aesculapius (*CSIR* 85) is found
in Chesters Museum; this is from Carrawburgh (*Procilitia*), (*63*) In addition to
the inscriptional evidence, the small bronze figurine of Aesculapius (*64*) found
near Chichester, West Sussex, is also of interest.

Gallic and Germanic healer-deities were sometimes identified with Apollo
the Healer, as at Glanum, a Graeco-Roman city in southern Gaul. The site
was originally a sanctuary where a health cult was dedicated to the god,
Apollo-Glan. It was shared by the goddess of health, Valetudo. However, such
syncretisation did not happen in the case of Aesculapius, whose special powers
may have been difficult to combine with that of Celtic deities.[49] Continuing
archaeological excavations at Glanum are focusing on the extensive cult wells.
Recent excavations have uncovered a Roman forum, a theatre and thermal
baths, with a dedication by Agrippa in 27 BC to Valetudo.

Also in Gaul, some 35km north-west of Dijon, in the early first century
AD, the shrine of the Gallo-Roman goddess Sequana in her capacity as a
goddess of healing, was established in a little wooded valley where the River
Seine arises from its source. Large numbers of sculpture were found, consisting
of 278 carved from wood and 391 in stone. Some were depicted bearing gifts,
others were anatomical depictions. In addition there were 300 votive offerings
made of metal, mainly eye plaques and torsos. Those made of wood were

carved from the heart-wood of oak and beech-wood, before the first century AD. There were models of rib-cages, viscera, carved human heads (sometimes multiple) and a recognisable hernia.[50]

In the early stages of the site, the votives were deposited in a *favissa*, or ritual pit. The waterlogged sediments in the spring preserved the wooden objects in anaerobic conditions, enabling their survival for 2,000 years. From the Roman period, evidence was found for the existence of a temple at the site, and it was here, on the walls, that the votives were probably displayed. Similarly, at the Source-de-la-Roche in Chamalières (near Clermont-Ferrand in France), more than 2,000 wooden statues and ex-voto parts of the body were found in a thermal spring. They were more Romanised in form than those from the source of the Seine. One of the heads was depicted with an empty eye-socket, perhaps suggesting blindness.[51]

Among other sculptured and inscribed stones of medical interest from Roman Britain, the presence of Mars, albeit conflated with epithets from native deities, seems to have been of particular importance. He was possibly first introduced to Britain by Roman soldiers. Such inscriptions, although not directly medical, are associated with health and medical care by their allusions to the fertility of human beings, of animals and of the earth, and, furthermore, to human welfare, nurturing and motherhood. Mars Alator, 'the nourisher', is found at South Shields,[52] on an altar from Cockburn Street, a little west of the fort. The deity also appears on one of a series of silver-gilt votive plaques from a shrine near Barkway, Hertfordshire,[53] now in the British Museum.

At Caerwent two dedications were set up to Mars Lenus,[54] whilst at Chedworth, Webster proposed the existence of another shrine to that god.[55] However the inscription, on one of the crudely cut votive reliefs, is uncertain. The healing deity is plainly attested at Trier in Gallia Belgica, now in Germany, where a more important shrine to Mars Lenus is known.[56] By the fourth century AD an entirely British aspect of Mars was known as Nodens, attested at Lydney in Gloucestershire, for Nodens possessed a healing shrine at this Romano-British temple site. His specialism in healing was attested by inscriptions, anatomical votives, finds of offerings of pins, bracelets, rings and toilet articles, together with representations of his cult animal, the hound (*colour plate 27*). It was also apparent in the 1930s excavation undertaken by archaeologists Sir Mortimer and Tessa Wheeler,[57] when they discovered, as further discussed below, a temple-site whose plan resembled the sanctuary of Aesculapius at Epidaurus. This was furnished with fine stone buildings, a guest-house, baths, an *abaton* for incubation or sacred sleep, and a well-appointed temple.

A hound cared for the child Aesculapius and is often shown as one of the god's attributes; it is perhaps pertinent that Diana also had a hound. Furthermore, in a local context there may well have been an identification with the 'Cotswold' hunter-god, Apollo Cunomaglos, meaning Apollo Hound-Prince.[58] Nodens is equated with Mars on three votive plaques from

Lydney,[59] as well as on the bases of two statuettes found at Cockersands Moss near Lancaster where he may have had another shrine.[60] Other hounds are figured on votive plaques from a site in Clwyd, suggesting that Nodens was also worshipped in North Wales.[61]

The temple complex of Nodens at Lydney resembled the same basic plan as the Aesculapian temples at Epidaurus, Cos and Athens, where the sanctuaries possess a prominent temple with an *abaton* (*65*). As in ancient Greece, the

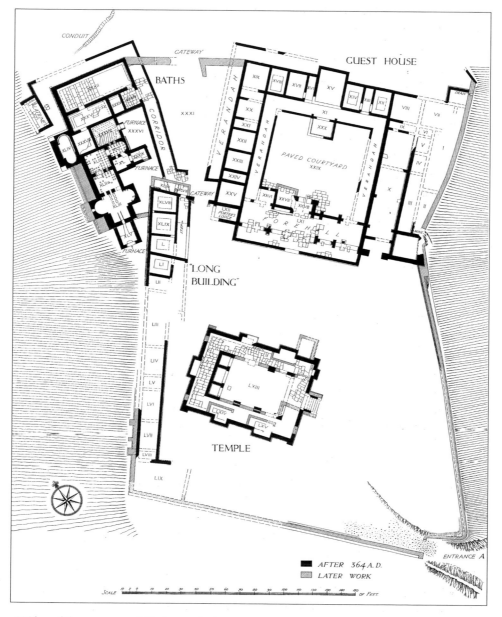

65 Plan of the sanctuary of Nodens at Lydney

135

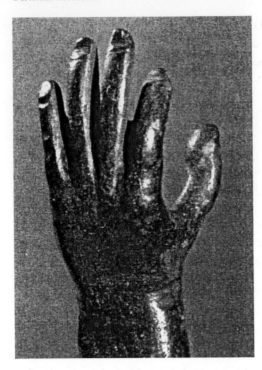

66 The votive hand showing deformed fingernails found at Lydney

abaton at Lydney may have been used for *incubatio* or temple sleep. The god would have appeared to the supplicant in a dream and after giving instructions, healing would follow, according to ancient belief. Alternatively, the patient may have been given certain instructions which were so cryptic that they required an interpreter (*interpres*), perhaps a priest residing at the temple. There is, indeed, evidence for such a person at Lydney; his name is Victorinus and he was named on the mosaic floor, now lost.[62] Although in temples of Aesculapius the lick of serpents is usually associated with healing, the lick of dogs was also curative.[63] At Lydney no representations of snakes have been found but there are a number of hounds in bronze or stone. Other sites where dogs were associated with Aesculapius are found at Epidaurus, Rome and the Piraeus, the port of Athens.

One of the most important anatomical ex-votos to be found in Britain is also from Lydney. Dr Gerald Hart[64] discusses the earliest example of specific therapy in iron deficiency, with reference to the small bronze forearm and hand found at the temple site.[65] In his opinion the spoon-shaped, concave finger nails (*koilonychia*) of the hand are diagnostic of iron deficiency anaemia (*66*). Although other scholars see such evidence as a possible metallurgical defect, the geological evidence at the site indicates that Dr Hart's diagnosis should be viewed positively. Although the bronze votive arm from Springhead offers no such diagnostic features as the Lydney example, other possibilities for the ex-voto are not hard to find. The earth at Lydney is visibly rich in iron. Indeed an intact iron-mine, dating to no later than the third century AD, was examined by archaeologists and is included in their report. A further anatomical votive from Lydney consists of a bone replica of a female figure. When found, it retained the bone pin which had attached it to the temple walls. Whilst it is possible that this votive represented a mother goddess, the small circle marking the area at her lower ribs could, however, signify a cyst or a 'lump', or even an enlarged spleen. In which case it, too, may be regarded as an anatomical votive with specific reference to the site.

The curative powers of iron may have attracted more than one sufferer from the symptoms of anaemia (enlarged spleen, extreme breathlessness, fatigue, loss of appetite, fragile bones) to take the waters or the earths at Lydney. It is easy to imagine that a rich folklore of remedies could have been broadcast far and wide once a few sufferers had found relief there, thus attributing healing properties to the site. The owner of the bone replica may have been another person with anaemia and she could have been suffering with unbearable pain associated with an enlarged spleen caused by the disease. Another scourge that caused much suffering among ancient peoples and which also caused anaemia was the presence of helminths, or intestinal parasites; yet another, and certainly no less deadly, was lead poisoning. However, a palliative, or perhaps a cure for all these symptoms could have been found at Lydney. The temple site was well patronised, as testified by the rich architecture and mosaics with which it was once embellished. An inscription, laid in the *cella* in the second half of the fourth century, attests the popularity of the sanctuary. It was laid *ex stipibus*, from the offerings of worshippers. As mentioned above, the dream *interpres* was Victorinus; the priest (*praepositus religionum*) at Lydney was Titus Flavius Senilis, also mentioned in the inscription.[66] The mosaic is lost, but otherwise the temple is quite well preserved and the finds are displayed in the small museum on the site.

The hot springs at Bath (*colour plate 28*) may have been famous throughout the Roman Empire, although the only reference to the sanctuary in ancient literature comes from Solinus[67] who records the curious stone (Somerset coal) burnt on Minerva's altar there. The presiding deity was Sulis-Minerva, a conflation of the Celtic Sulis with the Roman goddess Minerva; she was endowed with the healing aspect of Minerva-Medica. The Great Bath on the site of the spring is the most abundant; it constantly delivers about a quarter of a million gallons of water a day at a temperature of 46.5 degrees centigrade. The water contains calcium, magnesium, potassium, iron, lead and strontium. The temple precinct and its range of baths were constructed within a few decades of the Roman conquest and continued in use for four centuries, although, during this time, changes and elaborations were carried out. People suffering from a range of diseases including gout, rheumatism and arthritis would no doubt have found relief from the pain of it at Bath. Both Galen and Celsus recommended spa therapy for urinary tract infections and Soranus used water treatment for obstetric and gynaecological disorders.

Although several inscriptions testify to the use of the baths, none particularly specifies a medical use. Two of the inscriptions are the tombstones of soldiers who, to modern eyes, died very young, before their thirtieth birthdays, from which we may infer serious illnesses. Lucius Marcius Memor,[68] a citizen from northern Italy, dedicated a statue base to Sulis in front of the main altar at Bath. He was a *haruspex*, an Etruscan term meaning 'gut-gazer', an interpreter of the entrails of sacrificial victims.[69] It is probable that he was on the staff of the sanctuary, performing a useful service for the sick and other hopeful clients. A sculpture which may be a depiction of Aesculapius with his parents, Coronis and Apollo,[70] is also of interest, but due to its worn condition recognition as such is uncertain. Votive finds from the sacred spring, apart from coins (a number of which incidentally depict Salus, goddess of health), were few but there are two examples of anatomical ex-votos. The first is a fragment of a bronze breast and the second an amulet of a pair of breasts carved from elephant ivory, an expensive material. The white ivory may be symbolic of a mother's plea for continued lactation and the amulet would possibly be worn whilst the child depended upon her for nourishment and perhaps was later given to the goddess, Sulis-Minerva, in appreciation and thanks – an ex-voto. Another small ivory breast was found at the temple at Harlow, Essex,[71] where a head of Minerva, perhaps from the cult image, in oolite limestone was also found.[72] A further bronze breast is known from Uley.[73] There were also three votive legs from this site and at the first-century Romano-British shrine at Muntham Court in Sussex, another votive leg was discovered.[74]

Also at Bath, several *patera*, six bearing scratched or punched dedications to the goddess, testify to drinking the sacred waters and to pouring libations. In addition to the few votives from Bath, more than 100 'curse tablets' were found, indicating that gods could injure as well as heal. The curses were inscribed on 130 lead plaques representing the acts of aggrieved persons who wanted to launch into complex procedures of divine vengeance against someone who had injured them. Their language provides both a popular conception of pathology and also contemporary ideas about the human body. The denial of health through loss of blood or limbs is a common formula, whilst for the theft of gloves Docimedis asks of Sulis that the thief lose his mind and his eyes. These texts, as appeals to divine justice, are more religious than magical.[75]

CONTINUITY OF HEALING CULT

Supplications were made not just to the gods of the Graeco-Roman pantheon and local native deities. The pursuit of healing was also carried on through the mystery religions. Continuity of sacred space and healing is attested widely throughout the Roman Empire. It is represented at the Asclepieion at Athens,

Pergamum, Paestum, Nemi, Bath, Lydney and at many of the other major and minor shrines already discussed above.

A shrine in Roman Egypt for the incubation cults of Isis in Canopis and Menouthis illustrates the continuity of the oracle into the late Roman and early Christian periods. Large numbers of pilgrims, many of whom were prominent people, were attracted to the sanctuary at Canopis. The cult of Isis at Menouthis was established in the late second or early third centuries AD. This is known from an inscription referring to the goddess and to her 'true oracular words'.[76]

Votive *stelae* dedicated to the goddess include such symbols as pairs of 'hearing ears'. Isis combined her functions as a healer-deity with that of goddess of fertility. Later, attempts by Cyril of Alexandria to replace the healing power of Isis with that of the miracle workings of the Christian saints, Cyrus and John, ensured continuity of worship at the shrine.[77] The cult–centre of Isis was destroyed in AD 484 and a Christian church was established there, with relics of the saints. Healing continued to be obtained by sleeping near the enshrined relics, in both the pagan and the Christian phases of the shrine; therefore, healing by incubation was practised.[78] The function of Christ as a healer was one of the reasons for the spread of Christianity. However, what most people really wanted from the gods, rather than philosophical discussion, was help with the worries of daily life, whether the chosen god was an aspect of one or more pagan gods, or whether it was the Christian god, or even an amalgamation of all of them.[79]

Recently, in Jerusalem, archaeologists located the pool of Bethesda (Roman *Probatica*) in which Christ healed 'a great multitude of impotent folk, of blind, halt, withered,…' (John V.1-15), and it is no surprise to learn that this is adjacent to a temple of Aesculapius. Evidence from the pottery and coins dates the final use of the pool to *c*.AD 614 and its filling-in to the ninth century.[80] At Dor in Israel an archaic Greek temple of Apollo, belonging also to the later classical period, was dedicated to Aesculapius. Here the healing cult continued into the late Roman period. A Constantinian five-aisled basilica was founded *c*.AD 350. This included a reliquary column which incorporated a stone fragment from Golgotha and the reliquary tomb of two healing saints buried together. The reliquary column was destroyed by fire in the late seventh century. However, it is of great interest to note that in the seventeenth century AD, in Salisbury Cathedral, on a plaque commemorating a surgeon who specialised in eye diseases, Aesculapius is remembered again, when his name is used as a synonym for the title 'doctor'.[81]

~6~

ROMAN DISEASES AND HEALING II
'MEDICAMENTS, CAUTERIES AND OPERATIONS'

The third part of the Art of medicine is that which cures by the hand
... Now a surgeon should be youthful or at any rate nearer youth
than age; with a strong and steady hand which never trembles, and
ready to use the left hand as well as the right; with vision sharp and
clear, and spirit undaunted; filled with pity, so that he wishes to cure
his patient, yet is not moved by his cries, to go too fast, or cut less
than is necessary; but he does everything just as if the cries of pain
cause him no emotion

Celsus, De Med. III

From the fourth to the first centuries BC, at several sites throughout
western and central Europe, cremation burials of warriors who were
possibly also surgeons have been discovered. Grave-goods demonstrate
Celtic interest in medico-pharmaceutical problems through which it may
also be possible to trace Greek or Hellenistic influences.[1] One of these graves
was found at München-Obermenzing (Bavaria) where a group of iron
surgical instruments included an unidentifiable haft, a trephining saw and
a rounded-off *tenaculum* (usually a fine sharp-pointed hook) with an eyelet
handle resembling a modern probe. Similar grave-goods were discovered
at two other sites in Batina/Kis Köszeg (Hungary), whilst at Pottenbrunn-
Ratzersdorf (Austria) further grave-goods included an iron skull-rasp and
roundels of bone. Moreover, palaeopathological evidence from these areas
demonstrates that trephination was performed as a result of head-wounds. In
view of the warrior society to which the objects belonged, this is no surprise.
The evidence points to the use of circular metal trephines but such instruments
would not have enabled other types of surgery than trephination. Although
surgical tools originated in the Classical Greek world, the technical advances
achieved by the Romans in engineering extended into the manufacture of craft

tools and instruments of all kinds. Roman surgical instruments in particular were of extremely fine design and workmanship and the standards attained were equal to Roman achievements in other areas of technology. In addition, surgical instruments and medical implements provide a rich source of information for contemporary medical conditions and practices. An important surviving text is the *De medicina* of Celsus, who flourished in the reign of Tiberius.

The manufacture of specific and recognisable Graeco-Roman medical implements and surgical instruments began early in the first century AD. From this time onwards, they were made and used widely. Nevertheless, because they were not available in large numbers, their use was not distributed evenly throughout the Roman Empire. Roman surgical instruments represent the concentrated work of careful, highly-skilled craftsmen. As with the cult of Asclepius, the proliferation of medical tools around the empire was chiefly due to the movements of the army. This was equipped with a (largely Greek) medical staff who would have carried their equipment, theories and expertise to the outposts and frontiers of the Roman Empire. Some instruments were made from iron, whilst others were of copper and its alloys, chiefly bronze and brass. These materials could be cast, forged or cold-worked. Roman blacksmiths knew the art of imparting carbon to wrought-iron in order to make steel (carburisation) and bonding was achieved with tin-lead solder.[2] Further improvements in the quality of metal did not take place until developments in metallurgy were achieved in modern times. However, in the case of blades, which required a strong material, Roman craftsmen usually chose iron. Galen informs us that the best steel for surgical knives came from *Noricum* (present-day Austria).[3]

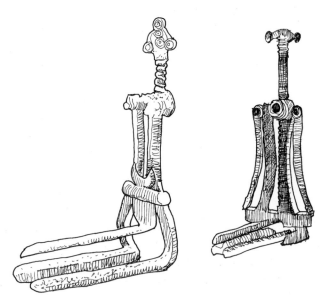

67 Right a) Graeco-Roman trivalve speculum from the Lebanon; b) *Far right* A vaginal speculum from Pompeii

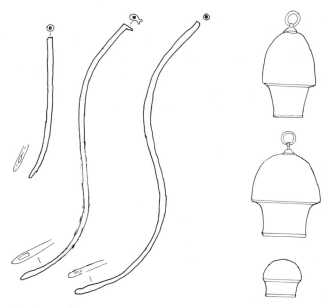

68 Left a) Male and female bronze catheters of the type found at Baden; *Right* b) Cupping vessels, *cucurbitulae*

Many surgical instruments were adapted for special procedures, such as the gouge found at Rimini,[4] which was of a type not previously seen. After comparison with a closely-associated trepanned skull, it was decided that this was a purpose-made instrument for performing trephination. Although the materials from which instruments were made varied, many types were of a uniformity which remained constant throughout the Imperial period and beyond. This is because once an instrument had established its use, the basic shape need not be altered. Vaginal specula (*67*) and rectal proctoscopes, male and female catheters, scalpel blades, artery and dissecting forceps as well as probes are a few examples of instruments which have retained their original forms until the present. This also applies to cupping vessels (*68*) before they went out of use in the twentieth century. Even in the case of scalpel-blades, although the size has changed, their form has not. However, the wider choice of materials that is now employed in the manufacture of them vastly improves their service.

WHAT CONSTITUTED A ROMAN DOCTOR'S KIT, OR INSTRUMENTARIUM?

Although Celsus was probably not a doctor himself, his writings in the *De Medicina* demonstrate that he was well aquainted with their habits and practices. He greatly admired many physicians, especially Hippocrates. In the surgical books (VII and VIII) the most frequently mentioned instruments are

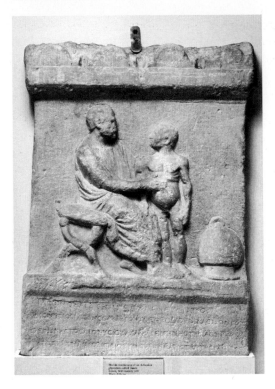

69 Marble tombstone of an Athenian physician called Jason, second century AD

surgical knives of various shapes and sizes as well as scalpels. In many of these the blade could be replaced when worn. The standard form of the scalpel had an iron blade and a bronze handle, which often terminated in a spatula for blunt dissection.[5] Celsus also refers to spring forceps, sharp hooks, needles, probes and cauteries, many of them also double-ended. In addition, cupping vessels (*cucurbitulae*) would have been required in various sizes. These were used in blood-letting and were also regarded as the symbol of a physician, as is apparent in the iconography of the 'Jason' relief in the British Museum (*69*). Archaeological evidence demonstrates that cupping vessels changed hardly at all from the late sixth century BC to at least the third century AD. They are found from one end of the Roman Empire to the other. However, cupping vessels are seen today as a sign of the practice of humoral medicine. It is interesting to note, therefore, that there has been no positive find of such an instrument in Roman Britain, leading to the assumption that humoral therapy, possibly, did not come to these shores.[6] Catheters, too, would have been required, most probably fairly frequently in view of the many references in the ancient sources to 'strangury' (retention of urine). Catheters were made from rolled strips of bronze; if these, along with blunt hooks, scoop probes and two sizes of saw are added to the above, then the portable kit of instruments that a doctor should carry about with him, as recommended by Hippocrates, is complete.[7] All the items would have been required in various numbers and in different sizes. Equipped with such a kit, the *medicus* would have been able to carry out a wide range of procedures.

However, some instruments not named in the *De Medicina*, such as rectal and vaginal specula, uvula forceps (*staphylagra*) and bone levers[8] are, nevertheless, present in the archaeological record, surviving because of either their size or their preservation in a favourable context. This indicates that in the early first century AD, at the time when Celsus was writing, such instruments either had not yet been developed, or else were not widely available. On the other hand, Celsus names some instruments that, so far, remain elusive as finds; an example is known as the spoon of Diocles, the *Diocleum cyathiscus* (Celsus, *De Med.* III. pp.319),[9] an instrument which was purposefully developed for the extraction of barbed arrow-heads.

The kit itself would have been carried in a specially made folding wooden box, such as the one illustrated on the tombstone of a Roman *medicus* from Athens[10] (*70*). In order to carry the slender and delicate probes safely, cylindrical bronze containers, similar to some modern pencil-cases, were made. In addition, specially compartmented bronze boxes, perhaps the precursor of the present-day 'doctor's black bag', were used to carry precious medical substances, such as drugs, unguents and powders (*71a*). Possible parts of such a metal box from Silchester in Hampshire, *Calleva Atrebatum*, may have held *materia medica*.[11]

According to medical writers in antiquity (Celsus, *De Med.*; Soranus *Gynaecia*; Paul of Aegina), practitioners in the Roman world had access to

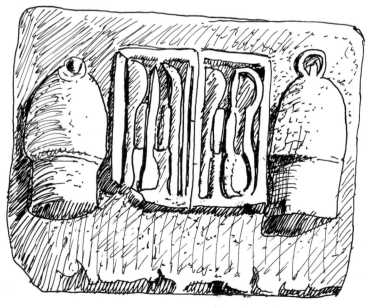

70 A marble votive relief showing a folding case of surgical instruments flanked by two cupping vessels. Roman, from the Asclepieion at Athens

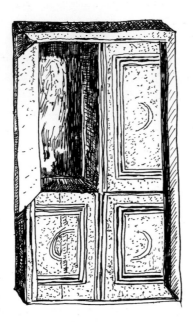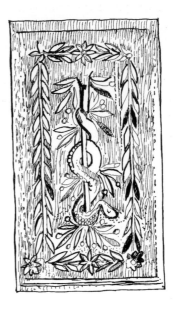

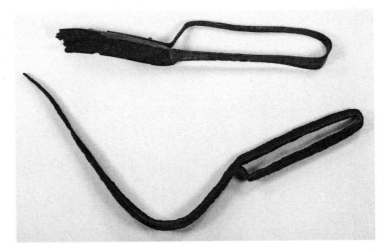

71 *Top* a) A typical bronze box with sliding lid and four compartments, used for the storage of *materia medica*; *Middle* b) An iron curette, combining a spatulate lever and sharp-rimmed scoop could have been useful in bone surgery; *Bottom* c) Iron needle: a domestic needle which could have been used for securing bandages

a wider range of medical equipment than those made wholly from metals. Organic materials such as wood, leather, woollen or cotton cloth, feathers and papyrus, which do not survive in the archaeological record, would have been used for splints, blankets, dressings and bandages. Even when instruments are made from metal, the preservation of them differs according to the context in which they are found. For example, if something is made from thin sheets of metal, such as rods, bronze vessels and containers, or sharp suturing needles and fine blades, it is often 'eaten away' by corrosion. It is surprising, therefore, in view of these difficulties of survival, that any such objects today remain extant. This disparity in the survival rate of different surgical instruments demonstrates the difficulty of even attempting to estimate how representative a picture we have, in the few instruments that have been successfully recovered, of the total number that were in use during the Roman period.[12]

Despite all these difficulties, several important collections of medical instruments have survived, such as those from Pompeii and Herculaneum, now in the National Museum in Naples. The British Museum (*colour plate 29*) and the Ashmolean Museum in Oxford also possess substantial collections. Recently more large finds have come to light. In addition, several museums possess small groups of instruments, or collections which are not a set but which come from a number of different sites, such as those in the Museum of London. Sporadic finds of instruments also occur in farmsteads and fortresses, testifying, perhaps, to the existence of travelling surgeons. Possibly the heads of households possessed one or two medical implements or surgical instruments with which to administer medical aid to family and slaves. However, it is generally the case that specific and recognisable Roman medical instruments are uncommon, and that they form a small and relatively insignificant category in a few museums. Often they are not displayed, and can be viewed only by special arrangement. Such a situation is found in museums abroad as well as in Britain and in some cases such objects have not yet received full publication.[13]

The context and provenance of an object are of primary importance in helping to establish a framework for its social history, manufacture and use. Sadly, however, in the case of surgical instruments such guidelines are seldom available. One of the reasons could be that their fine craftsmanship and particular associations, both from the past and of the present, make them highly attractive to collectors and treasure-hunters alike; perhaps more so than treasures of gold and silver. Thus, sets of Roman surgical instruments, such as that purchased by the British Museum in 1968 from a London antiquity dealer,[14] arrive in an almost 'anonymous' fashion, with few details of either the context or provenance. However, in this case as in others, as well as testifying to medical and surgical activity, the instruments themselves carry intrinsic information. Moreover, much of value can be learned from the analysis of attached corrosion products.

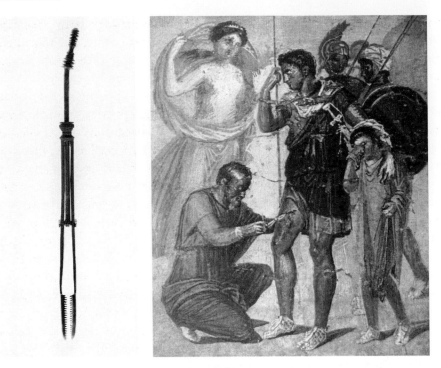

74 Left a) An unusual forceps held in the collection of the Ashmolean Museum, Oxford; *Right* b) An arrowhead is removed from the thigh of the wounded Aeneas with a cross-legged forceps; first-century AD wall painting from Pompeii

If surgical instruments are to provide insights into the societies, practitioners and patients for whom they were made, careful analysis of the means by which they were retrieved from circulation is essential. Where possible, this is best approached by an examination of the context of the find. Jackson[15] describes three such categories. Different processes are at work in each of them: site finds, grave finds and disaster finds. Individual site finds may represent ritual depositions rather than casual losses. Although in such cases reconstruction may not be possible, the possibility exists of gathering intrinsic information from the object itself. For example, the unusual forceps (74) assigned to the Roman Imperial period, held in the collection of the Ashmolean Museum in Oxford, is of great interest for the evidence it provides of the inventiveness of Roman surgeons, as well as the craftsman's skill for technological innovation. Of unknown context and provenance, it is a 'hybrid' of the staphylagra type and has an unusual plunger mechanism, allowing it to perform in 'profound and confined' locations.[16] Sepulchral finds, however, are slightly more informative, especially where the excavation technique has been carried out in a careful and sensitive way, as in the case of the first-century AD 'Doctor's Burial' at Stanway, Essex.[17] Several difficulties are inherent in this type of find. For example, the deposition of surgical instruments is a burial rite which does not extend to other Roman crafts. It is also unclear how much selection took place in the instruments which were deposited in the burial and, indeed, why these instruments in particular were chosen to be so consigned. Nevertheless, much of value was learned from the finds at Stanway and this is discussed further below.

Jackson's third category of find belongs to the so-called 'catastrophe' scenario. This includes instrument finds resulting from shipwrecks, volcanic eruptions and fires. It is possible for such unexpected and unlooked-for incidents to isolate and preserve whole assemblages of artefactual remains intact (albeit damaged) in their usual locations at the moment of disaster. However, even here there are caveats. It is important not to generalise the information gleaned from such a scenario beyond its immediate context. For example, shipwrecks do not represent a sealed context and neither do volcanic eruptions. At Herculaneum, the town was covered by a thick layer of tufa and the site remained sealed until the seventeenth century; however, looting was apparent at Pompeii which, covered by volcanic ash, was not totally sealed. In addition, the longer period of evacuation that was possible at Pompeii would have allowed people to escape, together with their possessions. Some of these could have been *medici*, or perhaps looters, carrying away medical equipment, as implied in the case of a man who was overcome whilst carrying a box of medical instruments away from the town.[18]

Conflagrations also belong in this category. Two recent examples, both involving extensive finds of instruments, await full publication. The first is in a house at the Roman town of Marcianopolis in Bulgaria, which burnt down in the mid-fifth century AD. It is said to include scalpels, shears, sharp hooks, handled needles, uvula forceps, bone levers, lithotomy scoops, rectal and vaginal dilators, as well as a trephining tool and an embryo hook.[19] The second example at Rimini, already referred to above, is the largest find of Roman surgical instruments yet seen. The site was excavated by Dr Jacopo Ortalli at Piazza Ferrari, Rimini, between 1989 and 1997. This 'house of the surgeon' in the Roman town of Ariminium was destroyed by fire in the mid-third century AD. The medical equipment included over a hundred instruments, drug boxes, melted glassware and instrument types not seen before. According to Jackson, 'this is the best evidence yet of what the equipment of a practising healer may have looked like'.

INSTRUMENT MANUFACTURE AND METAL ANALYSIS

In addition to information gathered from the context or provenance of surgical instruments, several other criteria need to be considered when examining new finds. These include the dimensions and details of style and the type and composition of the metal.[20] Once furnished with this information, it is possible to explore ideas regarding the function of the tool. Whereas craft tools or domestic implements are generally made from iron or bone, or a combination of both materials, surgical tools are made from iron and bronze, or copper and its alloys. Thus the differentiation of materials enables surgical instruments to be distinguished from other sorts of tools.[21] Analysis of an alloy can be used to identify and to link up sets and also to detect fraudulent copies, which will be betrayed by their high zinc content. Although some copies made in the later nineteenth and early twentieth centuries, in the Naples foundries, were not made to deceive but were 'polite' reproductions, gifts for souvenir-hunters, it is essential to discriminate between these two different types of *falsa*. Metal analysis can also be used to identify or confirm sets of instruments within an *instrumentarium*. Through such analysis it is often possible to ascertain the reason for the choice of a particular alloy used by the craftsman.[22] So far, named makers of instruments are unknown, neither is it clear whether they were specialists who dealt exclusively with surgical instruments or simply general blacksmiths. A few samples carry manufacturers' marks but at present these are insufficient to be of real use. However, a database of such marks with a record of differences in fabrics, style and decor would be helpful in the identification of regional workshops and instrument-makers.

By the second century AD, the healing centre at Ephesus in Asia Minor had become a sanctuary of some importance. The medical writers Soranus (*c.*AD 100) and Rufus (AD 70-120) were among its residents and the sanctuary was regarded as the hub of medical activity.[23] Annual contests were organised, with the results recorded on public inscriptions, a series of which survives. One of the events attested is a competition whereby physicians designed new medical instruments and attempted to adapt old ones to new uses. The discussions and sharing of new ideas would have been a stimulus to experimentation and innovation, leading to the development of improved surgical tools and, ultimately, to benefits for the patient. There would, perhaps, have been the inevitable tendency towards artifice or display on the part of some individuals. However, there was as yet no proper anaesthesia or knowledge of antisepsis. The Roman patient would have needed great courage or faith in order to undergo the procedures described in the ancient texts and attested to have been practised in the forms and manufacture of surgical instruments.

SUGGESTIONS FOR THE FUNCTION OF CERTAIN DECORATIVE MOTIFS FOUND ON ROMAN SURGICAL TOOLS

Nearly all Roman instruments were finely, even exquisitely, decorated whilst others, even when rather plain, were no less handsome. Some of the patterns used were simple striations; there were also abstract motifs such as diamond patterns or raised and incised rings, inlaid with silver or gold. The roughened surface would have enabled the surgeon to maintain a secure grip on the instrument, a necessity in all procedures undertaken. Whilst it was imperative for the physician to gain the confidence, consent and co-operation of the patient, this would probably have been a difficult objective to achieve where anaesthesia was unreliable and the treatment of infection was poorly understood. However, an interesting theory[24] suggests one of the ways in which such a difficulty may have been overcome. Physicians could have been enabled to gain their patients' trust and to persuade them that the risks of surgery were worthwhile by their choice of decoration on the tools that they used. In the modern world, advertisers of material goods effectively use secret signals and subliminal messages as a medium of psychological persuasion. Similarly, such devices may have been at work in the ancient world, where particular motifs on surgical instruments were symbols which carried associations and meanings to which both the surgeon and the patient were receptive.

Many of the decorations on surgical instruments were of naturalistic animal or vegetable designs. Among this group are three mouse handles (75) discussed by Jackson.[25] On the handle-ends, which are not completely identical, a mouse is depicted with great care. The animal is seen holding and nibbling what is probably a nut, between extended paws which are carefully depicted, as are the ears, eyes and pelt. The handles also carry inscriptions, not as carefully drawn as the mouse itself, an indication of their being of less importance. The finest of the handles is without provenance. However, corrosion products on this handle indicate an origin in Mediterranean lands. A further handle is in the British Museum and, according to records, probably came from the Artemision at Ephesus. The other one, now in the Römisch Germanisches Zentralmuseum, Mainz, has a vague provenance of south-west Asia. It was decided, after analogy with a grave-group of surgical instruments, which contained a similar handle, and also by qualitative analysis, that the handles could have had medical applications. They are considered to have carried a blade which was either a scalpel, a surgical knife or a razor. It is closely argued by Jackson that the inscription,

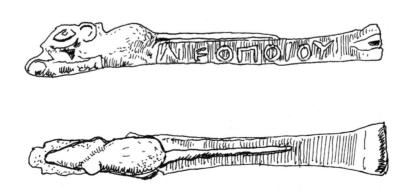

75 An inscribed bronze handle with a representation of a mouse on the terminal end

Hygeinos Kanpylios, signifies a temple official, a *neopoios*. In addition, through the presence of the mouse, there is a link to Apollo Smintheus, a healing deity revered in the eastern Greek world, whose cult animal it was. Jackson writes: 'it is not inconceivable that the Ephesian Artemision … was the original source of all the inscribed handles and that the sanctuary where they were found was that of the temple official named on them, Hygeinos Kanpylios … who may have been a healer and a medical teacher at the temple'. He would also have been well known to suppliants attending the temple.

Another interesting design seen on surgical instruments and other items closely associated with the human body is the bark and knot pattern, described by Bliquez[26] as the 'knotty limb' pattern. The pattern has been identified on approximately twenty-five surgical tools by specialists in the subject who are generally agreed that there was a connection between the 'knotty limb' pattern and the club of Hercules. Indeed, the design was seen as 'symbolising the power of the hero and the god himself'. The reason for the popularity of Hercules and his club as a motif on surgical tools is found in the traditions of his life. Famous for his strength, courage and endurance, he was also the universal helper and was frequently invoked as an averter of evil. The Hercules motif occurs mainly on instruments which are primarily associated with extreme pain, such as elevators, probes, needles, scalpels, retractors and possibly birthing hooks. However, it is not seen on the more benign items, such as spoons, ligulae and spatulae.[27] Baths and bathing are also associated with a medical function and it is no surprise to find allusions to Hercules in the *instrumentum balnei*, such as the bronze strigil from Reculver in Kent (*42*).[28] Another strigil inlaid with the labours of Hercules is found at Caerleon,[29] and a further one from a grave in Cologne also bears the pattern.[30] The motif is present, too, on bronze *unguentaria*, in which precious oils were taken to the baths, such as that from Pompeii.[31]

In the National Archaeological Museum in Naples, scalpel handles (minus blades) carrying the Hercules motif were matched with an old photograph (Alinari Pe.Ia. No.19087) depicting three such instruments with their blades intact; thus the connection between Hercules and Graeco-Roman surgery was confirmed by analogy. This was also confirmed by a retractor from Mainz, which again featured the 'knotty limb'. In addition to this there was a depiction of a lion's head, the former suggesting the club of Hercules and the latter the skin and head of the Nemean Lion – two attributes of Hercules in one instrument. Other connections between Hercules and medicine are found at a spring sanctuary at Deneuvre (Meurthe-et-Moselle) where two funerary *stelae* portrayed the god. At other sites in the Roman Empire, Hercules is seen in association with Asclepius. However, these few sanctuaries with connections to Hercules portray healing through faith and cult, whereas the instruments with the Hercules motif promote the influence of the god/hero into the realm of surgery,[32] thus giving the surgeon divine assistance in what must often have been supremely challenging work. The presence of an attribute of the god could have been experienced as a powerful apotropaic device by both the doctor and the patient.

A state of increased psychological sensitivity could have been achieved in the sick person by the administration of one of several drugs used to obtain altered mental states. Mugwort, *Artemisia vulgaris*, was a drug favoured for its hallucinatory effects. 'Dream states' were produced in which reality was perceived on a different level. Whilst under the influence of such a drug, the mental state of the patient would have been especially receptive to powerful symbols. The imminence of a deity who was seen as a 'paragon of endurance and resolute suffering'[33] would surely have been an inspiration to a person who, full of fear and dread, was anticipating surgery. *Artemisia vulgaris* is said to have been sacred to and beloved of shamans and, as such, was perhaps much used in rituals in the ancient world.[34]

SOME OF THE INSTRUMENTS AND THEIR USES

Trephination is one of the most ancient of all surgical procedures. A magical or ritual component is sometimes suspected. Those circular pieces of human skull-bone, dated to the prehistoric period, referred to above, may well have been excised for use as amulets. Skeletal evidence demonstrates that trephination was performed with a shell, a flint or a piece of obsidian.

Although the presence of trephines in the archaeological record is rare, a kit from Bingen-am-Rhein, near Mainz, in Germany, comprising two *modioli* and a folding handle is extant (*74*). At Colophon (Turkey) and Marcianopolis (Bulgaria) only a folding handle remains.[35] In addition, unprovenanced folding

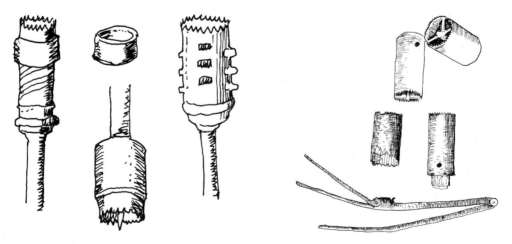

74 Left a) Two bronze trephines and the folding handle used to rotate them, from the large set of instruments found in a grave in Bingen; *Right* b) Variants of the cylindrical trephine, possibly in use in Greek and Roman times

handles may also be seen in the collections at the British Museum and the Berlin Antikenmuseum. In Britain, skeletal evidence demonstrates that trephining was practised from prehistoric times, throughout the Roman occupation and beyond;[36] however, no such kit is known in Britain. One reason for this is perhaps the friable nature of sharp-bladed instruments. In the Roman world there were valid medical reasons for carrying out trephination, as Pliny (*Nat. Hist.* 25.7.23) writes:

> … the experience of time has concluded that the disease causing the sharpest agony is strangury from stone in the bladder; next come diseases of the stomach, and after that pains produced by diseases in the head: these being the only diseases that are responsible for suicides

Apart from headache, which was an early symptom in many diseases, for example malaria, Pliny (in his reference to suicides) may also have had in mind painful mental states such as envy, paranoia, depression, hypochondria, or any of the other manias that are found in the ancient texts, associated with life in Republican or Imperial Rome. As well as its use as therapy for headache or epilepsy, or as a relief for intra-cranial pressure, trephination could also 'stop' a hairline fracture in the skull. However, according to Celsus, trephination was principally devised for the removal of diseased or damaged bone not only of the skull, but also of other parts of the skeleton, such as the breast-bone or ribs.

Many pages in Celsus are devoted to a discussion of cranial surgery. The main danger during or after surgery was fatality caused by damage to the coverings of the brain, or infection of the wound leading to meningitis, probably also fatal. For this reason Celsus recommended the procedure as a last resort. His description of the *modiolus* and the two types of trephine is clear (*De Med.* VIII.3). Regarding the actual operation, he claims that to saw through the bone was relatively easy, but warns of possible damage to underlying tissues. Where fracture of the skull was suspected, Celsus writes that it is first of all important to distinguish between the skull's natural suture and the fissure that could be caused by a fracture. The safest way to do this was to lay bare the bone and to apply ink over it. When scraped with a chisel, the crack in the bone would retain the blackness of the ink – presumably the natural suture-line would not retain the colour. Celsus describes two kinds of instruments. The first is a crown trephine, a circular saw with a serrated cutting edge, like a pastry-cutter. The other instrument was a solid-tipped drill. Bone is excised in two ways:

> If the damaged part is very small, with the *modiolus* which the Greeks call χοινεικίς, or crown trephine; if more extensive by means of trepans. I will describe the use of both. The *modiolus* is a hollow cylindrical iron instrument with its lower edges serrated; in the middle of which is fixed a pin which is itself surrounded by an inner

disc. The trepans are of two kinds; one like that used by smiths, the other longer in the blade, which begins in a sharp point, suddenly becomes larger, and again towards the other end becomes even smaller than just above the point. When the disease is so limited that the *modiolus* can include it, this is more serviceable; and if the bone is carious, the central pin is inserted into the hole; if there is black bone, a small pit is made with the angle of a chisel for the reception of the pin, so that, the pin being fixed, the *modiolus* when rotated cannot slip; it is then rotated like a trepan by means of a strap. The pressure must be such that it both bores and rotates; for if pressed lightly it makes little advance, if heavily it does not rotate. It is a good plan to drop in a little rose oil or milk, so that it may rotate more smoothly; but if too much is used the keenness of the instrument is blunted. Then, when a way has been cut by the modiolus, the central pin is taken out and the modiolus is worked by itself.

Celsus enters into much detail when describing the procedure for the operation and the subsequent care of the patient: 'As regards abstinence and food and drink at first and later, the same course is to be adopted as I prescribed for wounds, and all the more because the danger is greater when this part is affected' (*De Med.* VIII.4.19-22). However, the trepan, as already mentioned above, was not used exclusively on the bones of the cranium (*De Med.* VIII.2.3):

> ... But whatever is wholly diseased is to be wholly removed; if the lower part is sound, only that which is corrupt should be excised. Further, if there is caries of the skull or breast-bone or rib, the cautery is useless, and excision is necessary. Nor are we to listen to those who await the third day after the bone is laid bare before excising; for all cases are treated more safely before the inflammatory reaction occurs. Therefore, whenever possible at the same sitting, the skin is to be incised, and the bone exposed, and freed from all that is diseased. And much the most dangerous case is in the breast-bone, for even if the operation has been successful, complete healing scarcely ever results.

Celsus has more to say about inflammatory reaction at III.10.3, in a passage which gives a definition of the four cardinal signs of infection, well known to those caring for patients after surgery, even in modern times:

> Now the signs of an inflammation are four: 'redness and swelling with heat and pain' – *Rubor et tumor cum calore et dolore* – over this Erasistratus greatly erred when he said that no fever occurred apart from inflammation. Therefore, if there is pain without inflammation,

nothing is to be put on, for the actual fever at once will dissolve the pain. But if there is neither inflammation nor fever, but just pain... it is allowable to use hot and dry fomentations from the first.

The discussion of the use of trephination and the trepan provides an opportunity to illustrate one of the difficulties met with in the study of surgical instruments, briefly touched upon above. Whereas it is known from skeletal evidence that trephination was frequently performed, finds of the necessary instruments are few and there are none from Britain. Such a lack applies also to cupping vessels and vaginal specula. Despite their bulkiness few of these are found. At the other end of the scale, by comparison, small instruments, such as sharp hooks, surprisingly, have survived. In the archaeological world it is accepted that a lack of evidence does not necessarily indicate their absence. On the other hand, surgical operations for which the appropriate instruments are well known, are those used for removal of the uvula and for crushing haemorrhoids, known as the *staphylagra* and *staphylocaustes*[37] (75).

Surgical removal of the uvula is rare in modern laryngology; it is performed where there is swelling or elongation of the small organ caused by allergy or chronic inflammation in the throat. The operation involves cutting off the fleshy, cone-shaped appendage which is suspended from the middle of the soft palate. It has an important function in that it hangs like a curtain between the mouth and the pharynx and, with the root of the tongue, closes off the mouth cavity from the air-way of the pharynx when swallowing. Excision of the uvula is mentioned in the Hippocratic treatises and, although he does not specify the use of particular instruments, it is also described by Celsus (*De Med.* VII.12.3). In the Roman period it was possibly a common operation and it is comparatively well attested by finds of the appropriate instruments, some of which may have been used in Roman Britain. We do not now see the badly infected throats of the pre-antibiotic days, although given poor nutrition and unhygienic

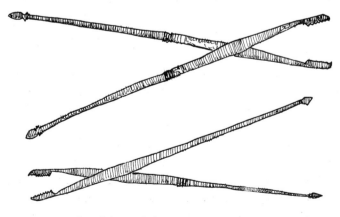

75 Two examples of the *staphylagra*

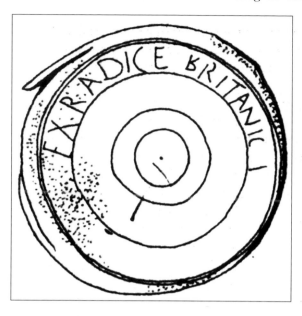

76 The lid from a jar found in the *principia* at Haltern; the inscription probably refers to the *radix britannica*, used as a cure for scurvy (after Guy de la Bédoyère)

conditions such a chronically infected and ulcerated throat is easy to imagine. Infected tonsils, too, would have been prevalent, especially in poorer communities. Celsus says that tonsils become hardened after inflammation (VII.12.2-4) and he recommends their extraction. 'Since tonsils are enclosed in a thin tunic, removal should be attempted by scratching round with a finger and drawing them out... although it may be necessary to assist this operation by seizing them with a sharp hook followed by excision with a scalpel'.

Preventative measures for these sorts of infections were evidently known, for Pliny (*Nat. Hist.* 25.6.19-21) writes that a certain herb, which he calls 'britannica' (76) (which may have been common scurvy grass, *Cochlearia officinalis*, found all around the coasts of Britain) was good for diseases of the mouth, throat and, in particular, quinsy (peritonsular abscess). According to Pliny: 'its juice keeps away quinsy for a whole year'. Britannica also cures scurvy of the gums. Thus, through empiricism the value of vitamin C was discovered, although it was not identified, of course, until a much later period in the history of nutrition. The plant would have been much valued in the Roman world, where poor oral hygiene and mouth infections caused much suffering. Ancient authors, including Celsus, recommended cupping and purging in preference to surgery, which was considered to be highly dangerous and to be performed only as a last resort.

In the Roman period, as now, the sufferer from quinsy, or any other suppurating condition of the mouth or throat, would have been chronically ill with high fevers, lassitude and a poor appetite. In the absence of antibiotics the potential for fatality, especially in young children, would have been high. The elongated uvula in such a sorely infected throat would be a flabby, oedematous nuisance, liable to cause choking and suffocation, and removing it was most probably the best thing to do. However, as with removal of the tonsils, even today, this was a hazardous procedure, with the possibility of fatal loss of blood and further infections, including difficulty with swallowing which would add to the patient's low condition, causing malnutrition and a slow recovery.

As an alternative to the radical surgery previously described, Celsus recommended partial removal of the uvula, simply by cutting off the tip, with a knife. The instruments carried in the standard *instrumentarium* would have been adequate for this apparently simpler procedure. Alternatively, 'if the tip is bluish-black and thick' the *staphylagra* was used to crush the neck of the appendage and then to twist it away 'until it becomes lifeless' – a method which, it was considered, would reduce the risk of haemorrhage.[38] Jackson reports that the use of the *staphylocaustes* is found in the late Hippocratic treatise 'De Medico' (I.63.5), and much later Aetius (II.IV.12) and Paul (VI.31) provide descriptions of the instrument. According to Jackson, a similar broad geographical range can be discerned for the cross-legged, toothed uvula forceps and *staphylagra*, to that of cupping vessels (though of shorter proven chronology). Indeed, Jackson's catalogue demonstrates that their use was widespread in the Roman Empire, with 'examples from Britain to Syria, and from Moesia to Cyrenaica'. Unfortunately, several examples have no provenance. The use of the *staphylocaustes* involved a different instrument and therapy. This instrument had capacious, hollow, spoon-shaped jaws, which could contain a caustic substance, 'the same as used for burning the eyelids... of a consistency not too liquid... lest it burn adjoining parts... telling the patient not to swallow but to remain with his mouth opened wide'. When this substance was applied to the scirrhous uvula, it would burn up and shrink.[39]

Paul of Aegina records the use of both the *staphylagra* and the *staphylocaustes* in the second century AD for removal of haemorrhoids. Two types of instrument can be discerned, with either straight or bowed arms. The latter type may have been intended for use only in haemorrhoid operations, simply because the bowed-arm type would not allow such easy access to the throat as the straight-armed type. The possession of these two instruments would increase the repertoire of procedures which the Roman surgeon could offer to sufferers from sore throats or piles. In his catalogue, Jackson[40] includes twenty-six medical instruments, all of similar design. The toothed *staphylagra* was probably the most useful of the two types. Nine are in Britain and of these six are of unknown context and unknown provenance. Exceptions are his No.1 from Caerwent, now in Newport Museum, No.20, which is from Colchester and is now in the British Museum and No.23, also from Colchester and in Colchester Museum. All these finds with known provenances can be assumed to have been used for their particular purposes in Roman Britain. The type from Italy, now in Bristol City Museum, is complete and in good condition (77), although the instrument may have been a recent arrival and perhaps was not present in

Roman Britain. The six items of unknown provenance, one of which (No.11) is in the Townley collection in the British Museum, were also probably not from Roman Britain. The other instruments in the illustration from left to right include a double-handled sharp and blunt hook, bifurcated hook and a scalpel handle. Of a different sort is a *coudée* type from Littleborough on Trent.[41] This instrument would serve the same purposes as those described for the *staphylagra*. It would also be possible to use this instrument for the removal of surplus skin from the eyelid in the operation for ingrowing eyelashes (trichiasis). The artery forceps excavated at Silchester, *Calleva Atrebatum*, although badly distorted, was complete with its locking ring.[42] This, too, could have been used for the eyelid operation in addition to other procedures.

SITES IN BRITAIN WHICH HAVE PRODUCED MEDICAL INSTRUMENTS

So far in this chapter much of the evidence has been derived from Roman sources dating to the post-conquest period. However, the two expeditions of Julius Caesar to Britain in 55 and 54 BC doubtless left a mark. Caesar was accompanied, among others, by his personal physician who would certainly have possessed a medical kit. Another focus of interest here concerns the Druids. Caesar and other ancient writers provide information concerning the functions and learning of this ancient priestly caste. They are recorded as officiating in both Britain and Gaul and would have exerted powerful influences on the native population. Almost a century of contact between Southern Britain and the Roman world followed Caesar's visits before the invasion by Claudius in AD 43. It is possible that in the Celtic lands a pool of shared

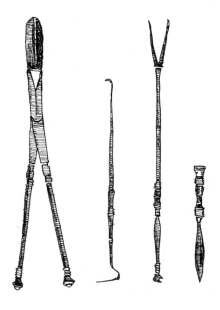

77 A set of instruments from Bristol City Museum. From left to right: forceps for applying caustic *(staphylocaustes)*, combined sharp and blunt hook, bifurcated sharp hook, scalpel handle

medical knowledge had already existed, an idea that is reflected in Jackson's comment, '... there may have been few novelties brought to Britain by the Roman Army'.[43]

At the sacred site at Stanway, near Colchester in Essex, a funerary site for a group of Britons who died in the late Iron-Age and early Roman periods, was excavated intermittently between 1987 and 1997 by the Colchester Archaeological Trust. In 1997 the cremated remains of an adult, who had been interred with a set of surgical instruments, were recovered. This is the first 'definite and properly excavated ancient British medical kit from Britain'.[44] The grave was dated to about ten years after the Roman conquest, raising pertinent questions about medical practice in Britain at this time and relationships between native Britons and Romans (*colour plate 30a*).

Although other objects of great interest were found in the burial, the interment of the instruments suggests that the buried person was a doctor who had practised surgery. The kit is of great rarity and importance and has attracted a considerable amount of interest in Britain and elsewhere, from specialists and the general public alike. It was viewed by the writer in November 1997, when on loan to the British Museum. Initially it was the ancient board game that excited the greatest attention. This established the grave as a burial of high status. (Another gaming set was included in a burial from Welwyn.)[45] The cemetery where the doctor's grave was found was about a mile away from Gosbecks Farm, where a theatre associated with a temple site is known.[46] Four large funerary enclosures were excavated at the cemetery at Stanway and this was a satellite burial (*colour plate 30b*). Among other finds was a dinner service of eleven Gallo-Belgic vessels, an amphora, a ceramic flagon, a samian bowl, a copper-alloy pan and a brooch. Judging from the finds in this and adjacent burials, it is possible to infer that this was a wealthy family group.

When found, the medical instruments were seen to have been placed on and around the board game which lay open with its blue and white glass counters in a position of play. The cremated remains were placed in a heap on one half of the board. Also included in the burial and displayed in London with the medical kit were eight somewhat enigmatic rods, four made of copper alloy and four of iron, each about 30.5cm in length. Three of the rods were laid end to end to overlap the board and the others were placed on one side. These were accompanied by metal rings which were about an inch in diameter. The question arose as to whether this was another type of game, or perhaps the rods and rings were associated with the instruments and the practice of medicine? The most favoured idea, at present, is that the rods were related to divination which, in the ancient world, often possessed an affinity with medicine. Rods of a different shape and later in date are known from Chelmsford.[47] Because everything else in the grave appeared to have been intact and complete when buried, a small surgical saw which was found broken into five pieces and carefully placed in a tight group near the centre of the board, is especially curious.

Crummy[48] suggests that the burial could have been that of a Druid, a caste whose members were masters of traditional lore, including healing, in the Celtic world. A further native aspect of the grave is attested by the presence of a metal strainer of the same type that was present in the Welwyn grave.[49] In the strainer from Stanway, however, a plug of various pollens was found, the dominating one (comprising about 95 per cent of the plug) was a member of the Artemisia family. The hallucinogenic properties of *Artemisia vulgaris* have been discussed above but, it is emphasised, at the present time the exact species found in the Stanway kettle has not yet been identified.

The instruments themselves are more Celtic in form than Roman, six of them being of one-piece iron with knobbed terminals. This Celtic feature is reminiscent of the terminals on the fire-dogs from Mount Bures, near Colchester[50] and also on linch-pins, sword-hilts and belt-hooks.[51] Buried in the middle of the first century AD, the set of instruments found at Stanway is the earliest surviving group from anywhere in the ancient world. The trephines and surgeon's instruments found in the Celtic graves at München-Obermenzing and Kis Köszeg, to which reference was made above, although very fine, possessed a limited functional range. While most of the Stanway instruments are subtly different from the standard forms acquired in the first century AD there are, nevertheless, related features. The instrument-find itself can be said to consist of a modest but complete set of the basic tools of ancient surgery,[52] an *instrumentarium*. In total there are fourteen instruments: one small knife, two one-piece iron scalpels, two combined sharp and blunt hooks (one iron and the other copper-alloy), smooth-jawed copper-alloy forceps, pointed-jawed iron tweezers or forceps, a set of three iron-handled needles graded in size, a copper-alloy scoop probe, a double hook and a small iron saw with a handle of copper alloy and bone.

Although there are similarities to Roman instruments in the Stanway kit, for example, in the shape of the scalpel blades, as single-piece iron instruments they are substantially different. A Roman scalpel would have had a bronze handle and an iron blade which could be replaced when worn. In the Stanway scalpels the blades are dissimilar, the first having a cutting edge and the other a straight, leading one. The handle ends on the three other iron instruments in the set probably terminated as solid-handled needles. These are also un-Roman, being made from single pieces of iron, instead of possessing the Roman-style socketed bronze handle which could then take replaceable iron needle tips. In Roman medical literature, it is possible to find many uses for these instruments, from the removal of embedded foreign bodies to suturing wounds and from bone surgery to puncturing haemorrhoids. They were also used for delicate work on the eyes, such as removal of cataract. In addition, some of the instruments, such as the needles, could have served as cauteries.

The person buried in the grave, who was probably a native Briton, seems to have been in contact with Roman doctors and was familiar with some of the precepts of classical medicine, arising, perhaps, from those earlier pre-conquest expeditions to Britain.

At Silchester, in addition to the bronze artery forceps complete with its locking ring to which reference has already been made, other finds from the Roman town are also of interest.[53] These include long narrow ointment spoons, a small bronze balance and arms, as well as stone palettes for grinding medicaments and rolling pills (as illustrated in *colour plate 31*). There was also a spring-forceps with pointed jaws and a combined smooth-jawed forceps and a square-ended forceps of bronze. All these instruments would be suitable for fine and delicate work. There are probes, too, and a *ligula* of fine quality, its stem inlaid with silver wire.[54] Part of a bronze instrument container is also present in this group. The excavator suggests that these could well have come from a surgeon's house in the Roman town, or from a *taberna medica*.

The instruments at Corbridge may be the group seen by Eric Birley, uncovered south of the main east-west road and seen and verified by a surgeon from the College of Medicine at Newcastle. They consist of several pieces, including three combination handles for holding scalpels. The first has a blade of steel at one end with a leaf-shaped spatula at the other which could have been used for blunt dissection or cauterisation. The second example is broken at both ends. The third scalpel is the most interesting in this set. It has a bronze spatula at one end and at the other are the remains of a steel scalpel blade surrounded by bronze solder, keeping it attached to the handle.[55] Also in this collection are three handles for surgical knives. They represent the two different methods whereby blades are attached to the handle, detachable or fixed as described above with reference to the Stanway set. Other instruments are tongue depressors and probes. Both the *specillum*, a plain rod of bronze which tapers to two blunt points, and the *spathomele*, belonging to a separate group of probes, are present at Corbridge. The spatula-probe, as with other instruments in this set, would be useful in a number of situations. The *cyathiscomele* we have already met above at Stanway. Here two types are represented. The first type has an angle in the middle and the second has the spatula formed into an elongated spoon. *Ligulae* were used for extracting ointments from *unguentaria* and balsams and powders from bottles of different sizes; the Corbridge collection has six of these.

According to Gilson,[56] 'the Roman cautery was used for almost every part of the anatomy, to treat a variety of infections, diseases, lesion, trauma … as a bloodless knife to destroy tumours'. In the National Museum of Antiquities of Scotland, Edinburgh, a collection of Roman surgical and medical instruments is displayed. The group included four spatulate objects identified as cauteries, all different. They were at the sale of a private collection and therefore a foreign provenance is a strong possibility. However, sited at Cramond was a Roman fort and civil settlement so a local context need not be entirely dismissed. Although in Hippocrates (Aphorisms VII 15.1) the cautery was to be used as a last resort, Celsus has many uses for the instrument. Jackson[57] describes three broad categories: the staunching of blood, the destruction of diseased tissue, or the removal of healthy tissue to give access to underlying structures. Of further interest are two bronze sharp hooks, one from Housesteads and the other from South Shields.[58] Parallels have been found elsewhere on Roman sites in a medical context, for example at Bingen in Germany. No record has been found for the Housesteads example and no hospital has been found at South Shields, despite the presence there of other medical objects. Blunt and sharp hooks are frequently mentioned in Latin medical texts. They are used, *inter alia*, for dissection, for raising blood vessels and for traction in midwifery.

At Norwich a number of surgical implements are listed in the accession records and in the Sites and Monuments Record. One of the most interesting is the bronze instrument from Hockwold-cum-Wilton, Norfolk. It was examined and its details were subsequently published by Dr Calvin Wells.[59] The site from which it came has produced a number of votive objects and probably included a sanctuary. The instrument consists of a handle 90mm in length. From the handle springs a curved cylindrical shaft. Wells decided that this was a uterine sound, much used in classical times. Galen and Soranus both refer to them. Tertullian (*c*.AD 160-*c*.225) writes of a 'bronze sound with which a secret death is inflicted. They call it the 'εμβρυοσφακτης 'foeticide'. According to Wells this instrument would be well adapted to such a use. When placed beside his own uterine sound, the two instruments are seen to be almost identical – as seen in the illustration (*78*).

In the Museum of London a fine assortment of medical instruments is displayed (*79*). They are not a set but come from a number of city sites. The only publication of them so far available is a brief appearance in the London Museum Catalogue published in 1930 and reprinted in 1946.[60] The context of the find is not given in every case.

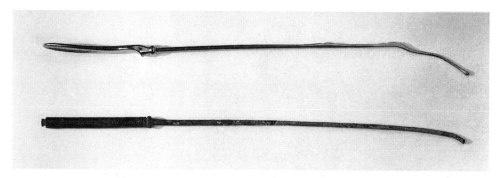

78 The uterine sound from Hockwold-cum-Wilton (*below*), set beside a modern type (*above*)

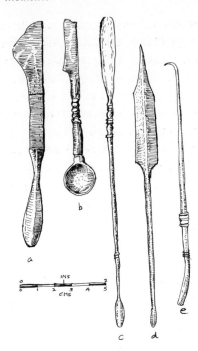

79 Shown here is a selection of
instruments from various London
sites: (a) is in the Museum of
London; it is the only scalpel to be
found complete with its blade in
Roman Britain;[61] (b) a spoon-bladed
spatula of bronze from Tokenhouse
Yard; (c) a spoon-bladed spatula
of bronze from Finsbury Circus;
(d) another spoon-bladed spatula of
bronze from the Royal Exchange;
(e) a double-edged instrument
comprising a sharp hook and a
probe, of unknown provenance.
Redrawn from Liversidge, 1968

EYE SURGERY, COUCHING CATARACTS

... But there are grave and varied mishaps to which our eyes are
exposed; and as these have so large a part both in the service and
amenity of life, they are to be looked after with the greatest care ...

Celsus, *De Med.* VI.5.6

The most famous example of an eye-injury in the ancient world is that of
Philip II of Macedon, who suffered a horrific wound at the seige of Methone
in 354 BC. Extensive damage to the eye-socket in this case was attested after
his skeleton was found in a family grave at Vergina, where the bones have been
positively identified. Accidental injuries to the eyes and adjacent tissues were
common, as were other sorts of eye-infections, ailments and defects. These
are widely reported in Greek and Roman medical texts. They also feature in
the Greek medical papyri from Roman Egypt. Blindness, then as now, partial
or complete, would have been a serious handicap, especially for people with
families to care for. Significantly, blind beggars, too, are frequently met with
in ancient texts.

Although complicated surgery was undertaken on the eyelids and the tissues
surrounding the eyes, the only operation that intruded into the eye-ball itself
was that performed for cataract (*80*). However, the lens at this time was wrongly
assumed to be the seat of vision. The aim of the operation was to reduce the
opacity by the insertion of a bronze needle with a tip that was 'pointed enough

to penetrate the eye, but with a rounded tip and not too fine… to be inserted straight through the two outer tunics at a spot between the pupil of the eye and the angle adjacent to the temple', (Celsus, *De Med.* VII.7.14). The cataract was '*couched*', (the word comes from the French *coucher* meaning 'to push down'). Celsus says 'if the lens sticks there the cure is accomplished. The needle is then drawn out and a pad of soft wool soaked in egg-white is placed over the eye' – an interesting juxtaposition of matter. Celsus recommended the procedure as a last resort, being well aware that the operation did not always successfully restore sight and also that as a result of it the patient could lose the eye through damage or infection. Although the anatomy and physiology of the eye were

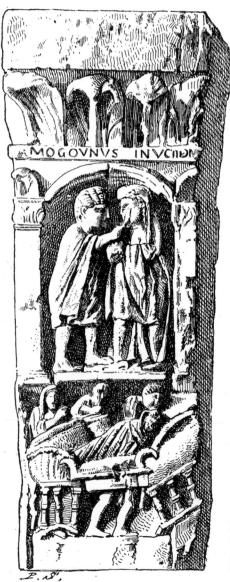

80 A Gallo-Roman physician on a funerary monument. The centre panel may show eye surgery

165

poorly understood, in some patients, particularly those with short-sightedness, there may have been a degree of success once the clouded lens was removed. Such success would have confirmed the incorrect idea that the lens and the cataract were separate bodies.

> For this disease there are many salves devised by many inventors, and these can be blended even now in novel mixtures, for mild medicaments and moderate repressants may be readily and variously mingled. I will mention the most famous.
>
> <div align="right">Celsus, <i>De Med.</i> VI.6.2</div>

Celsus writes extensively about afflictions of the eyes and, although references are found in several places throughout his work, for the most part they are located in Bk VI.6-7. The extent of the problem of eye disease in the ancient world is apparent in the number of conditions he describes. It is also attested in the inscriptions on oculists' stamps; some prefer the designation 'collyrium' and generally the terms seem interchangeable. In this chapter, however, the traditional term 'oculists' stamps' will be used, although it should be noted that these were mainly the property of eye doctors, whereas collyrium stamps were used by healers.

OCULISTS' STAMPS

The small stone blocks bearing Latin or Greek inscriptions, cut in retrograde, first came to light in France and elsewhere in the seventeenth century. Obviously of great antiquarian interest, their relevance to eye-medicine was soon established. In contrast to the religious dedications to be described below (chapter 8) the inscriptions on the stamps attest a more 'scientific' approach to medicine. They were formulated to treat a wide range of disorders and diseases and, in addition to the recipe, or prescription, the name of the person who formulated the salve is also engraved on the stamp. Empire-wide, more than 300 collyrium stamps are known (Jackson, 1996a, p.2241) with the majority coming from the north-west provinces; possible reasons for the distribution of the stamps is now discussed.

In addition to their testimony concerning diseases of the eye and their treatment and, as well as the names of the formulator of the salve, oculists' stamps are also archaeological evidence for regional differences in medical practice.[62] The lack of such finds in the Levant and most especially in Egypt, where the incidence of eye disease has always been high, is 'as impressive a piece of negative evidence as the heavy concentration in the north-west is a positive one'.[63] A number of theories have been put forward in an attempt to explain this curious, even absurd, situation. One suggestion is that the stamps have a military origin. This idea is founded on the endorsement by Galen (XII

786K) of Axius, the *opthalmikos* attached to the *Classis Britannica*, in which Galen refers to him as a specialist eye-doctor.[64] The theory of a military origin for the stamps is also based on the contexts of the finds, for several collyrium stamps are from forts and fortresses. Another suggestion attempting to explain this extraordinary concentration of stamps is the 'fiscal' theory propounded by Künzl.[65] This has its origins in the close correspondence between the Roman tax region of the four Gauls with the distribution of the collyrium stamps. Movement away from the four Gauls would have been discouraged by taxation and this is seen as a possible concession to eye doctors in the Mediteranean provinces, perhaps as a form of 'protectionism'.[66] However, this theory is yet to be supported by documentary evidence.

A further suggestion[67] is that the distribution of the British stamps indicates a medical system different from that found elsewhere in the Empire. In Britain, where the system was probably adapted to the requirements of a largely rural-based population, the doctors may have formed guilds, or *collegia*, in urban centres and from there they could have travelled to outlying parts of the countryside. Moreover, Jackson demonstrates that twenty-seven of the thirty stamps are found in places situated along the routes recorded in the Antonine Itinerary[68] this lends support to the idea of the itinerant eye-doctor, thus making sense of the need for pre-packaged, ready-to-use sticks of eye-salve, as well as of the stamps themselves (*81*).

Interpretation of the context and provenance of stamps is complicated further by the high potential for their misuse. The stamps, with their curious inscriptions and miniature size, are attractive tactile objects and as such they are eminently portable.[69] The owner of a stamp could have used it for personal identification, like a signet ring or medical visiting card.[70] Jackson suggests that such stones could also have been endowed with magical or supernatural virtues for use as a charm or amulet. He cites the example of the stamp from Goldenbridge, Co. Tipperary in Ireland (*RIB* 2446.28), found in a dyke where human bones were also present. Although the stamp could well have been taken to Ireland by its original owner, whose purpose was medical, it is also possible that its presence there was completely unconnected to the practice of medicine.

Peripatetic eye-doctors may have practised medicine in baths, markets, fairs, theatres and amphitheatres, or wherever large groups of people gathered (as was also the case in medieval and even in early modern times). Sacred places should, of course, be added to the above list, for stamps have been found in the vicinity of the temples of Sulis-Minerva at Bath and of Nodens at Lydney. At Wroxeter two collyrium stamps (*colour plate 32*) as well as votive eyes (*51*) were found (*RIB* 2446.14 from the *macellum* and *RIB* 2446.18 from the débris of the basilica). The latter stamp, unusually, is circular in shape. Stamps found on the basal interior of samian ware[71] (*RIB* 2446.25.i-ii, cups, and iii, a plate) possibly designate the property of the practitioner (*colour plate 33*). The cup or

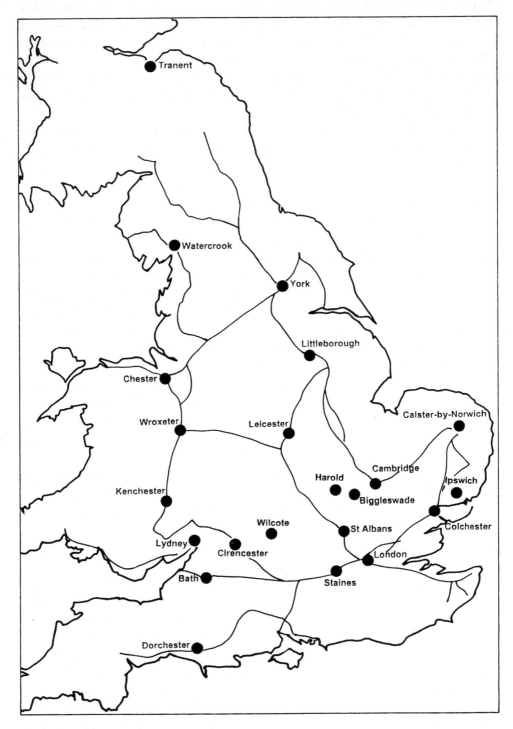

81 A sketch map showing the distribution of British collyrium stamps in relation to the roads of the Antonine Itinerary. *After Jackson*

plate was to be used as a container for mixing or holding special ingredients. When filled it was probably not considered necessary to see the stamp inside the vessel because the contents would be easily identified by sight or smell. For example, in the case of 'Lucius Iulius Senex's saffron salve for granulation of the eyelids' (*RIB* 2446.15) from Colchester, the ointment would have been bright yellow. Saffron is also a vital ingredient of the eye-salves known as *crocodes* and *apalocrodes*, mentioned on six out of the thirty eye-stamp prescriptions described by Jackson.[72]

Finds of stamps at villa sites, for example *RIB* 2446.13 from Lansdown, Bath, *RIB* 2446.17 from Shakenoak, Oxfordshire, and *RIB* 2446.31 from Whitton, Suffolk, support the idea of the itinerant eye-doctor who would visit people in their own homes, or elsewhere. As stated elsewhere in this book, in Roman society the *paterfamilias* acted as both the family and the estate physician and was often in possession of sets of medical equipment which included instruments. Such a set could have included a collyrium stamp. However, on a large estate 'the master as doctor' might also employ either a resident or an itinerant eye doctor, especially at times when eye infections were rife. The collyrium stamp *RIB* 2446.9 from the temple site at Lydney Park may well indicate that there was an eye-doctor in residence. This could also be the case at the sanctuary of Sulis-Minerva at Bath, as well as for those found at Abbey Yard and Wroxeter public baths (*colour plate 34*).

Although it is said to be from a military site, the stamp *RIB* 2446.5 found at Watercrook is not from the fort but from the east *vicus*, found in an unspecified 'phase three' context, dated to the Antonine period.[73] The oculist, Publius Clodius, who worked in the vicus at Watercrook and is named on the stamp, may well have been a Greek. The stamps from Dorchester, Colliton Park and London Upper Thames Street, riverside building[74] possibly indicate the home of a healer, or *taberna medica*. The prescription *penicillum* (or *penicillem*) *ad lippitudinem* (for inflammation of the eyes) is marked on two British stamps, one from Colchester, *RIB* 2446.8 and the other from Cambridge, *RIB* 2446.22, whilst *penicillem ad impetum lippitudinis* (at the onset of inflammation), *penicillem ad omnem lippitudinem* (for every kind of inflammation), and *penicillem post impetum lippitudinis* (after the onset of inflammation) are found on a further eleven stamps, three of which are from Britain, including the newly found Staines stamp.[75] According to Celsus, *lippitudo* was a common and troublesome complaint in the Roman Empire as a whole. He refers to it as a chronic inflammation following trachoma but it can also mean simply 'running and discharging eyes'. It is easy to imagine the rapidity with which the infection would spread, assisted by itinerant eye-doctors, literally like 'wildfire'.

Suggestions of itinerant eye-doctors practising in crowded places and in peoples' homes or in forts or fortresses are interesting in themselves, less as demonstrating cures for eye disease then as perhaps suggesting the cause of them. There is no doubt that eye-doctors as peripatetic *circuitores*, carrying their equipment around with them, would be ideal transmitters of such highly contagious diseases as conjunctivitis (*lippitudo*) and trachoma (*aspritudo*). There was some realisation that infections could be 'caught'. This is demonstrated by the evidence of the Vindolanda tablets[76] where soldiers suffering from *lippitudo* were segregated both from the wounded and the sick men. However, real knowledge of antisepsis was inadequate and conditions in rural areas would certainly favour the spread of any infections, possibly to epidemic proportions, as discussed above. This would apply particularly to infections of the eyes, especially in situations where sticks of collyria were used directly on the eye when they might just previously have been used on the eyes of another infected person, or even as a probe in a suppurating fistula.

It seems reasonable to assume, therefore, that what started as a different system, related to the needs of a largely rural-based population served from urban centres, became the direct cause of perpetuating the contagion. An increased demand for eye-salves would lead to a growth in their manufacture and use and eventually to more finds of eye-stamps. The idea that a greater prevalence of eye disease existed in the north-west provinces, or that more treatment was given in that area than elsewhere, does not now seem quite so absurd. For Celsus the word *ophthalmia* meant running, watery and inflamed eyes, otherwise called conjunctivitis and trachoma. Opthalmia today is a collection of symptoms involving the eye, including iritis which is only seen by examination with a special 'slit' lamp. This condition could not have been diagnosed in antiquity. 'Rheum' is a thick, white discharge, which when it is dry and sticky gives rise to pain. Celsus informs us that Hippocrates used blood-letting, medicaments, wine and baths for these conditions. Moreover, he is critical that little explanation is given for either the reasons or the frequency of these remedies, perhaps a slight hint against the practice of humoral therapy? For pain in the eyes Celsus recommended bed-rest, with clystering of the bowel on the second or third day of the illness.

So far, some of the therapies available to patients in the Roman world have been discussed. In the following chapter we come closer to the Roman patient when we discuss their physical remains. Lastly (in chapter 8) some of the practitioners will be identified. From Italy, Asia Minor and elsewhere in the Empire the writings of physicians have come down to us. In Britain, however, medicine was different. Here the full impact of humoral medicine may not have been experienced outside the ambit of the Roman Army.

∼ 7 ∽

MEETING THE ROMAN PATIENT

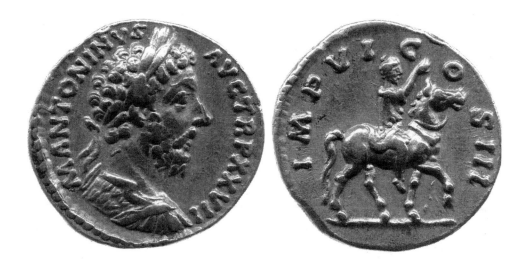

81a Marcus Aurelius spent much of his reign under the shadow of the plague, which arrived in Rome in AD 156/7. We know him more intimately than other emperors because he recorded his inner thoughts and feelings in his 'Meditations', written whilst he was on campaigns and published after his death. In AD 169 he appointed Galen as court physician, thus this most high-profile patient is tended by the most high-profile Roman physician. According to his writings Marcus Aurelius is known to have suffered severe chest pains and for these Galen prescribed various Theriacs, whose chief ingredient was opium. Although Galen was well-aware of the dangers of addiction, there is no evidence that the Emperor became addicted. On the subject of pain Marcus writes: 'For times when you feel pain see that it doesn't disgrace you, or degrade your intelligence, doesn't keep you from acting intelligently or unselfishly (Meditations 7, 33); he would nevertheless have found relief in the medication, for he was troubled by debilitating chest pains and the plague whilst on his death bed. [1]
Courtesy of British Museum

WHY PALAEOPATHOLOGY?

Palaeopathology is the study of the diseases of ancient people; it is pursued at various levels of experience. Palaeopathologists, sometimes known as

171

physical anthropologists or anatomists, come from a wide variety of specialities, such as archaeology, anthropology, anatomy, ancient history, biochemistry, biology and genetics. In archaeology we are interested in more than the classification of ancient diseases; the chief concern is with the general health of past populations, their way of life, their nutrition and their longevity. The integration of archaeological, biological and cultural data greatly illuminates any present knowledge of past societies.

Ethics and legislation governing human burials may vary from one country to another, but (with the exception of some infamous cases), it is universal for peoples to treat their dead with humanity and respect. This same sensitivity extends into studies of human remains. In all cultures the passing of human life is marked by rituals which reflect the religious beliefs of the deceased. Burial sites and funerary practices often provide insights into such beliefs, and also into the social structures of ancient societies.

The study of the diseases of our ancestors involves the macroscopic and the microscopic examination of ancient bones and, where it exists, soft tissue. Even cremated bone, albeit fragmented and distorted, provides useful data concerning both the individual and the cremation itself. Bones from burials, however, are much more useful, although these, too, have their problems, in that soil conditions affect the preservation of bone. The most important factor in this respect is soil acidity. Under some acidic conditions, bone may not survive at all. I refer, for example, to the Romano-Saxon cemetery at Mucking, Essex, where the only evidence for human skeletons was staining of the soil in the graves. The major causes of death in antiquity would have been caused by infectious diseases which affect soft tissue only, leaving no marks on the skeleton. However, soft tissue seldom survives and much of the total burden of disease and injury in a population is invisible to the palaeopathologist.

GENERAL REQUIREMENTS FOR THE PRACTICE OF PALAEOPATHOLOGY

The study of human skeletal remains requires expert knowledge of osteology, anatomy and dentition. Skills in recording standardised measurements of various bones are needed in order to determine the age, sex and stature of the deceased. Bones are examined for abnormalities due to injury, disease, occupation and congenital anomalies (*82*). This macroscopic examination is in contrast to the scientific methods which require the use of the microscope.

Before the advent of scientific analysis, the estimation of sex and age at death in adult skeletons was an art rather than an exact science, and in many ways it remains so. For, although such assessments may, on occasions, be problematic, real expertise comes with practice and experience. Where possible the skeletal remains will be photographed in the position in which they were initially discovered, before removal for further investigations. X-ray studies

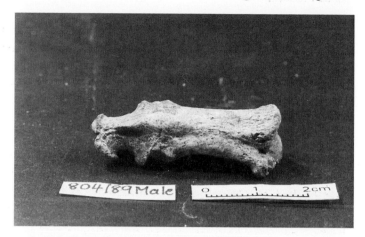

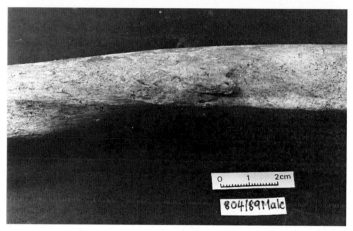

82 Two examples of healed trauma in the right humerus of a male skeleton at the second-century villa site at Sherston, Wiltshire

complement the osteological examinations. These are best performed by experienced technicians with adequate equipment and radiation monitoring. It is often made easier and more accessible by collaboration with an interested radiologist from a friendly local hospital. Any remaining soft tissue is collected in suitable containers for histological examination.

In addition to the parameters described above, it is also possible to gather information concerning contemporary surgical practices from the study of human remains. This includes trephination and methods for setting and healing fractures. Often an individual's occupation is apparent in the skeleton. This is seen in the *condyles*, or bony swellings, which develop for the attachment of muscles. A well-developed musculature requires firm anchorage points and such bony swellings evolve accordingly.

Initially it is necessary to know what is normal in order to be able to understand what is abnormal, and to be able recognise the pathological. Some diseases, such as tuberculosis of the vertebral column (Potts disease),[2] and rickets in children, or osteomalacia (the adult form of rickets), anaemia and neoplasms, are easily recognised in bone. Others, such as the destructive joint diseases, which directly affect the bone and its coverings (gout, for example), are also visible to the naked eye.

A skeleton found at Cirencester[3] dating from around AD 150 showed partial destruction of several joints, plus small cavities in the cortex of long bones; more than fifty of these lesions were present throughout the limbs. This was diagnosed as a classic example of gout.[4] Wounds and injuries, too, where they leave tell-tale signs on the skeleton, add much to an individual's personal history. For example, the multiple well-healed bone injuries found at Cirencester, indicative of deliberate aggression, show no signs of medical intervention. Thus a window is provided on the history of the Roman population in the late fourth century AD.[5] In rare cases, cause of death may be apparent from the skeletal evidence. For example, a Roman *ballista* bolt was found embedded in the spine of an individual from Maiden Castle, Dorset. For the bolt to have become implanted in this way it would have had to pass through the aorta, the main artery of the body, and death would have occurred from internal bleeding within minutes.

In addition to using skeletal material to learn about individual occupations, diseases and ancient medical practices from bones, it is also possible to see evidence for congenital abnormalities. These may be due to an inherited genetic fault, such the haemolytic anaemias which result in obvious bony changes. The achondroplastic dwarf was not hidden away in antiquity, as witnessed in the ancient world in art and literature. At Rome dwarfs held positions of high honour, such as in the courts of the Emperors Tiberius and Alexander Severus; Mark Antony, too, was known to have retained them as counsellors.[6] Spina bifida is known in Roman Britain; examples are found at Cirencester and Poundbury where several people are seen to have suffered from this anomaly.[7] At the Roman villa at Keston in Kent there is another such case.[8]

Replacing the traditional methods used in palaeopathology, several laboratory investigations are now available. These include electron microscopy examination, chemical and biochemical checks, blood grouping and DNA testing. In recent years new techniques in molecular biology, radio-carbon dating, X-radiography and CAT scanning (which allows the examination of tissues such as mummified or frozen remains without their destruction) offer the possibility of recovering further, and much more precise, data than was formerly possible. For example, the co-operation between forensic science and archaeology has brought about the reconstruction of a living face on a dead skull. New scientific tests continue to be developed allowing further possibilities for research into human skeletal material.

One example of a relatively new scientific method is the technique, developed in the late 1980s, known as Polymerase Chain Reaction (PCR), which allows extremely small quantities of DNA from bones, tissues and teeth (or any other type of organic material) depending on its burial conditions, to be used for analysis. The major use of ancient DNA in bones is for sex differentiation and aging, as well as the study of diseases and kinship analysis. DNA is one of the most valuable substances to be recovered from archaeological remains, but it is extremely fragile and easily contaminated, both in transit to the laboratory and also whilst in use there. In most circumstances, however, bone seems to provide an excellent, protective carrier for it. However, all these laboratory tests are expensive.

The principle of PCR is that the extraction of a minute amount of DNA can be used as a template for more and more copies of that DNA to be made. Detection in the skeleton of disease-causing bacteria or pathogens may reveal, for example, *Plasmodium falciparum* (one of the causative agents of malaria), *Mycobacterium tuberculosis*, or bacteria of the genus *Trepona*, which cause leprosy, yaws, and endemic and venereal syphilis. It is possible that further work may look at the mounds of ancient Syria and the Near East, where a 'potential gold-mine of genetic information exists'. In this area some of the first bacterial pathogens to have caused diseases in early urban man may be discovered.[9]

However, the use of PCR may yet serve another purpose: infection leaves lesions on bone from which it was always possible to hazard a diagnosis. Research shows that organic material is able to remain in bone for thousands of years. This has implications for palaeopathology. It means that when a bone becomes infected during life, under certain conditions, it is possible for the organism to remain present after death and to live on in the grave. On finding traces of a specific pathogen through microscopic examination, the original conjectural diagnosis of the bone lesion may, or may not, be confirmed. This type of laboratory work is of utmost archaeological value. It could well be of use in helping to determine the role played by bacteria and viruses in shaping history,[10] for example in identifying the specific cause of a plague, or the geographical course of syphilis – the latter is a subject of continuing controversy.

ASSESSING THE AGE AND SEX OF SKELETONS

DNA studies[11] are also used for 'sexing' immature skeletons; an example comes from Roman Ashkelon,[12] on the southern coast of Israel. Here the skeletal remains of 100 babies were discovered in a sewer beneath a bath-house which had been built in the fourth century AD, over the debris of earlier Roman villas. Lamps decorated with erotic images had originally been found there. When viewed together with a Greek inscription, 'Enter, enjoy and…', which the excavators found in the bath-house, it was suggested to them that the building could also have served as a brothel, as was common in the Roman Empire. The skeletal remains were of one- or two-day-old infants. They showed no signs of disease or malformation; therefore this was suspected to be an example of the practice of infanticide. It was decided to test the bones for gender identification by molecular methods. Stringent controls were observed in the laboratory and, to avoid testing the same individual twice, left femurs only were analysed. There is ample evidence for infanticide of females in Graeco-Roman society,[13] so it was a surprise when it was found that, compared to that of the females, almost three times as many of the total assemblage that could be reliably analysed were males.

Regardless of possible explanations for this event, the example illustrates one of the ways in which molecular biology is used to further the advance of archaeological research. The study at Roman Ashkelon demonstrates the use of DNA analysis in human skeletal remains where there is a need to obtain evidence for the resolution of archaeological questions. However, such tests are too expensive for all but the most especially interesting cases. The 'hands-on' methods of analysis for estimating age and sex in skeletons, as used by palaeopathologists, is a specialist subject, concerning which many books, journals and articles are readily available in libraries and bookshops. Some are listed in the bibliograpy; below is a brief introduction to a few of their precepts.

SKELETAL GROWTH

Age at death in young children is relatively easy to estimate because early growth and maturation follows a predictable sequence. Long bones in the foetus are formed of cartilage, represented by rods or blocks of this substance, or, in flat bones, sheets of membrane, resembling in shape the mature bone. The next stage in development is calcification caused by the deposition of lime salts in the cartilage or membrane. Bone cells or osteoblasts enter the calcified cartilage together with osteoclasts which help to remove it. The bone cells then proceed to lay down new bone in place of the cartilage, which becomes absorbed; this is ossification. It takes place *in utero* at about the eighth week after conception.

The skeleton grows quite rapidly both during intra-uterine life and in the first years of infancy. By measuring the long bones of a perinatal infant it is possible to determine its age to within two weeks. The shaft of the bone is the diaphysis. The ends contain a centre of ossification; these are the epiphyses. Each epiphysis is joined to the diaphysis by a layer of cartilage known as the epiphysial cartilage. This gradually becomes replaced with bone, by the process described above. At about the age of eighteen years the epiphyses and diaphyses are completely fused into a single bony structure, but, as long as some epiphysial cartilage remains, growth in the length of the bone is still possible.

Unification of the epiphyses occurs between the ages of seventeen and twenty-three years and is the criterion by which subject-age in young adults is established. Rarely, in over-activity of the pituitary gland, the unification fails to take place and the result is a condition known as gigantism, or acromegaly. In this condition, the bones of the face, skull, hands and feet, too, tend to be very large. On the other hand, it is possible for bone-growth to be slowed down by malnutrition or disease. If, whilst the bone is growing, the individual is subjected to any adverse influence, such as nutritional deficiency, childhood disease or severe emotional stress, it is possible for the process of active proliferation to be disturbed and for the growth cartilage to remain dormant for an indefinite period of time, depending on the cause. This may be a short, acute illness such as pneumonia or enteritis, or it could be the result of a period of famine, or protein starvation. Growth begins anew with the individual's recovery, but, as a result of the period of stress, a transverse line of dense calcification is left in the shaft of the bone, marking the place of arrested activity. These 'bone-scars', or Harris lines, are detected by radiography.

Similarly, lines of extra enamel (dental hypoplasia) and pits or grooves can occur on the teeth of juveniles. These, too, are assumed to mark out periods of illness or dietary stress. Like the Harris lines found on bones, they remain on the teeth in adulthood as a permanent record. Although such measurements have been demonstrated to be of practical use in studies of mummified material, other scholarly viewpoints need to be considered. Some researchers[14] claim that there are no certainties regarding Harris lines and dental hypoplasia, that they are not yet fully understood and that more study is required before such parameters can be reliably used in studies of the health of past societies. Although it may be possible to obtain an impression of age at death from the unification of the epiphyses, a more reliable assessment can be made through observation of the eruption of the teeth, for these follow a predictable sequence. Each individual has two sets of teeth, consisting of the temporary teeth of childhood, twenty in number, followed by the permanent set of thirty-two. The eruption of both sets follows a regular order. The earliest permanent teeth to appear are the first molars. They project from the gums behind the second, temporary molars. Others erupt in turn and the permanent set is complete by about the age of twelve, except for the third molars or wisdom teeth, which generally appear between the seventeenth and twenty-fifth years, or they may never erupt but remain buried in the gums. From the sequence of events described above, it follows that it is possible to estimate the age of a child's skeleton from the eighth week of conception to the twelfth year of life.

The most sexually dimorphic part of the adult skeleton is the pelvis, the difference being related to biological reproduction. The pelvic girdle consists of the right and left innominate bones plus the *sacrum*. The innominate bone is a large, irregular, flat bone which, in the child, consists of three parts separated by cartilage. In the adult these parts are fused together, but their separate names are retained to enable description. The uppermost bone is the ilium, the part on which one sits is the ischium and the anterior part is the pubis; the joint between the two is the symphysis pubis. The three bones unite and take part in the formation of the large cup-like cavity on the outer surface of the bone, the acetabulum, into which fits the head of the femur, thus forming the hip joint. The angle below the joint, the sciatic notch, is more open in the female. Another reliable indicator is the presence, or otherwise, of foetal bones in the pelvic area. The skull also has noticeable differences. In males the ridges on which the muscles moving the head and lower jaw are attached, are usually more prominent than those in females. Differences also occur in the size of the teeth and in some races the jaw-bone is definitive. The presence of particular types of grave-goods, or clothing, may also indicate male or female sex.

The male pelvis is long and narrow, the male skeleton being generally larger and heavier than the female; it follows that the female pelvis is broader and lighter. All the so-called differences enumerated above are flexible because many powerful influences affect the skeleton's formation and development, including heredity, occupation, disease, style of living, diet and environment. The dominant influence of one or other of these factors makes a difference to the individual skeleton. However, there is considerable overlap between the ranges of variation. In some cases, for example, when whole bodies are found in archaeological settings, such as the bog bodies or the Neolithic 'iceman' discovered in the Austrian/Italian Alps in 1991, assessing the sex is not a difficulty. However, none of these are from a Roman context; even so-called 'Lindow man', from Lindow Moss, Cheshire, belongs to the late Iron Age.

In more mature skeletons, as with the assessment of age in infants, the teeth are also prime indicators of age. This would be based on the level of wear on the molar teeth. The degree of wear and tear on the skeleton itself is a useful parameter, too. Bones change throughout the life of an individual. After the fusion of the epiphyses, adult bones continue to change with age, but the changes do not occur on a regular basis, as they do in the initial development. These changes occur in the microstructure of the long bones. Bone cells, osteoblasts and osteoclasts, as before, bring about a remodelling of the bone. In this process bone is continually removed and replaced in response to loading and stress. This leads to the formation of Haversian canals. These systems are detected by microscopic examination of a thin, transverse section of dense bone which is seen to be mapped out into circular districts, each having a central hole or canal surrounded by a number of concentric rings, or lamellae. They are plentiful in young people but in the elderly they become greatly reduced in number.

Other indicators of age are the appearances of the symphysis pubis joint, and the sacral surfaces, which change throughout life. In young adults the underlying surface of the pubis joint is deeply grooved, often with about eight intervening ridges criss-crossing it from front to back.[15] This joint is the body's principal load-bearer; the strains on it throughout the life of the individual cause the ridges to become less well defined as time passes. In females the stresses and strains of childbirth also act on these surfaces. Age at death is difficult to estimate in adults because skeletons vary so much, according to genetic inheritance as well as to the influences already enumerated above. In most cases the sex and health of an individual as well as the economic status all determine the rate at which that person ages. Longevity and height in adults are parameters of primary importance also because they can be used in assessments of the nutritional status of a population.

POUNDBURY

The excavation between 1966 and 1978 of more than 1,000 skeletons from the Romano-British cemetery at Poundbury, located outside the walls of Roman Dorchester, *Durnovaria*, resulted in a detailed and comprehensive report on the human remains.[16] The write-up includes a résumé of burial practices, the diet and nutritional status of the population, including diseases of malnutrition, infectious diseases and lead accumulation, congenital conditions, evident difficulties in childbirth, degenerative bone and joint diseases, parasitology, diseases of old age, and anaemia. Anaemia at Poundbury Camp, which is also the subject of two separate papers,[17] is discussed below.

ANAEMIA AT POUNDBURY CAMP

Anaemia is a deficit of red blood cells or haemoglobin in the blood; it is the most frequent blood disorder encountered in children today. This fact alone is sufficient to prompt an enquiry as to what was the situation in the past. Anaemia is another condition that is easily recognised in ancient skeletal material. The skull of an individual who had suffered from anaemia would show two types of visible bone lesion, each diagnostic of the condition. First, cribra orbitalia appear as sieve-like openings in the roof of the orbital fossa. The perforations begin as pinpricks but may increase in size to produce much larger lesions, so that underlying trabeculae become visible. As the marrow hyperplasia continues, similar lesions appear in the vault of the cranium. This is known as porotic hyperostosis, a term reflecting the two-fold effect that the increased size of the bone marrow has upon the bone itself. Porotic hyperostosis may also appear on the frontal, parietal and occipital bones. It is caused by the deficit in red blood cells, which stimulates the marrow to try to increase the manufacture of red cells (haemopoiesis), thus causing bone displacement.

Iron-deficiency anaemia is caused by dietary factors, parasitism, malaria or lead poisoning. Whilst the two former causes were studied and their possibilities were not dismissed, lead poisoning was considered to be the most likely cause of anaemia in Roman Britain. Lead is absorbed into the bloodstream through ingestion, inhalation or topically – through the skin. Lead levels were studied at Poundbury Camp[18] and comparison was made with the largely contemporaneous population at Cirencester, where incidence of anaemia and lead levels had been studied by Waldron in 1966. Stuart-Macadam concluded that at least one third of the juveniles had anaemia during their lifetime, but it was not possible to make statements about the acquisition of the disease during adulthood. The most likely cause seems to have been the extensive lead technology developed by the Romans. Lead was mined in Britain and was used for a variety of functions. In terms of producing anaemia, conditions at Poundbury and Cirencester were about the same; workers at the lead mines in the Mendips could also have lived in these areas. In this respect these are the two most extensively studied areas; we do not know about the rest of the population of Roman Britain.

The research team concluded that anaemia at Poundbury Camp was most likely to have been caused by a deficiency of iron in the diet. Parallel causative factors may have included parasitism, infectious disease or lead poisoning. At Cirencester similar instances of cribra orbitalia and porotic hyperostosis were found with male predominance. Wells[19] suggested that women preparing food were able to keep up their levels of protein intake by 'filching choice morsels' from the stew-pot and that this would have given them some protection from anaemia. The report concluded that the incidence of anaemia at Poundbury Camp was about average for prehistoric populations in general and similar to that seen at Cirencester.

DENTAL HEALTH AND POSSIBLE TREATMENTS

Although teeth are the hardest material in the human body, and as such are easily recoverable from archaeological contexts, the extent of dental disease in the Roman Empire is not well known (*84*). A few specific reports are available and by and large these speak well of the dental health of Roman populations. However, these conclusions are, of necessity, only partial. Furthermore, they are not borne out by the literary evidence from the first-century physician, Scribonius Largus,[20] nor by the writings of Celsus, or the wit of Martial. Nevertheless, at Herculaneum one researcher (see below) writes that 'the condition of the teeth of the ancient Herculaneans was excellent'.[21] In Britain, finds of teeth at Poundbury, Chichester and York demonstrate a remarkable lack of caries. Periodontal disease, too, was not considered to be extensive and tooth-loss was not high. However, tooth-loss among women at Cirencester was found to be 56 per cent more than that seen in men despite their life-span being, on average, three years less. Wells suggests[22] that poor oral hygiene among females may have been the cause of this, but perhaps, tooth-loss in females is far more likely to have been due to the exigencies of pregnancy and childbirth?

At the Roman cemetery at Newarke Street, Leicester,[23] where the dental remains of twenty-seven skeletons, comprising twenty-four adults and three children, were examined, tooth decay in this population was slightly more than that found at Cirencester. Dental abscesses were present at all of these sites, and are also seen in other more random finds. Such abscesses would have been quite painful, especially when the subject attempted to chew food. However, despite all these variations, it is, perhaps, no surprise to find that

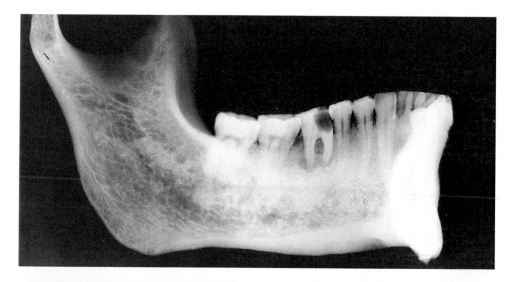

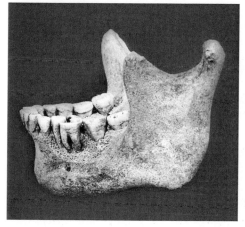
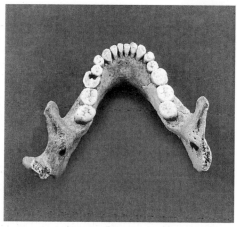

83 Photographs and an X-ray of the mandible of a male skeleton from the second century villa site at Sherston, Wiltshire, showing caries in the first left molar and an abscess exposing its roots

levels of tooth-loss and dental caries were significantly lower among ancient Romans than in modern populations.

Dental health has a nutritional factor. In all populations the presence of caries is closely related to diet. A low rate of decay implies that a largely meat and vegetable diet was taken, as against too much reliance being placed upon carbohydrate. It could also reflect the lack of sugar in the diet (sugar was not introduced into Europe until the Middle Ages when it was brought back from the Crusades). Honey, well known to Romans, would probably have been used much less then than sugar is used today. The lower incidence of dental disease in the Roman world need not imply the regular use of toothpicks, although these are frequently seen in archaeological settings and are known to have been placed on the dining tables of the élite.[24] Tooth-brushes are, of course, a modern phenomenon, but mouthwashes were well-known. The relatively low rate of calculus (tartar) as found, for example, at Cirencester, in contrast to that seen in modern mouths, is further evidence that a moderate amount of meat and coarse bread supplied much of the Roman diet. On the debit side, the abrasive effect of the slow chewing of coarse, stone-ground bread or porridge was extremely hard on the teeth and in some instances, such as those found at Poundbury, teeth were completely worn down.

Less well known are ways in which people may have cared for their teeth, if at all, and, indeed, what treatments were available when things went wrong. Dentistry was not separated from general medicine in first-century Rome and for Scribonius Largus it seems to have been of great importance, for he devoted some ten chapters of his famed *Compositiones* to the subject. But, as always, his main concern was with herbal medication – regarding which, he once famously said, 'such plants are the hands of the gods'. For Scribonius Largus surgery and cauterisation were the least acceptable forms of treatment. Indeed, to learn about dental surgery at Rome we should turn to Celsus. However, both of these writers were in favour of saving the affected tooth whenever possible. Scribonius' suggestion that dental diseases may have been fairly common in first-century AD Rome is, perhaps, corroborated by Celsus in his somewhat harrowing discussion of surgical measures (*De Med.* VII.12). When teeth have become loose due to gum disease or trauma, Celsus recommends the use of iron cautery to the gums. However, in Bk VI.9 Celsus tells of the treatment of toothache, and other dental conditions, using slightly more palliative measures:

> ... in the case of pain in the teeth, which by itself also can be counted among the greatest of torments, wine must be entirely cut off. At first the patient must fast, then take sparingly of soft food, so as not to irritate the teeth when masticating; then externally steam from hot water is to be applied by a sponge, and an ointment put on made from cyprus or iris oil, with a woollen bandage over it and the

head must be wrapped up. For more severe pain a clyster is useful, with a hot poultice upon the cheeks, and hot water containing certain medications held in the mouth and frequently changed. For this purpose cinquefoil root may be boiled in diluted wine, and hyoscyamus root either in vinegar and water, or in wine, with the addition of a little salt, also poppy-head skins not too dry and mandragora root in the same condition...

The belief that worms were the cause of dental decay was very real in antiquity; it lasted into the eighteenth century. Scribonius recommends a treatment (*Compositiones* LIII):

> ... it is necessary to fumigate the open mouth with the seed of hyoscyamus, scattered over charcoal, and to repeatedly rinse the mouth with hot water; for sometimes, as it were, little worms are expelled. And fumigations of warmed bitumen relieve the ache...

Suetonius (*Aug.* 79)[25] informs us that Augustus' teeth were 'small, few and decayed'; Scribonius' elaborate toothpowder, which was especially prepared for the Emperor, follows:

> Gather pellitory which is in seed and with many roots, then wash and dry it for one day; on the following day soak the hard parts in fresh brine; on the third day, after water has been pressed out, bring them together in a new earthenware pot; immediately afterwards they are to be placed between layers of salt and thoroughly cooked in the furnace of a bath-house; then partially burned over charcoal. Afterwards, the remainder is mixed with spikenard, which is pleasing. This then makes the teeth white, and makes them firm.

Octavia, sister of Augustus, was also known to use a dentifrice specially prescribed for her by Scribonius. It was meant to 'beautify and to strengthen the teeth' and was made by mixing barley flour with honey and vinegar, kneading it, and dividing it into little balls. Salt was then added to each ball which was afterwards burnt over charcoal, cleaned and mixed with spikenard to give it a good fragrance. Furthermore, we have the recipe for the tooth-powder used by Messalina, wife of Claudius; it possessed the following ingredients: '3 ounces of stag's horns burned in an earthenware pot and reduced to ashes, 1 ounce of Chios mastic, and 1½ ounces of sal ammoniac'.

Scribonius Largus seems to have mixed in court circles and it is no surprise to learn that he was an essential member of Claudius' invasion of Britain in AD 43. The length of his stay in Britain is not known, but further evidence for the early entry of medicine into Britain is seen in the surgical instruments, some of classical form, found in the Stanway burial (see chapter 6). In addition to his pastes and mouthwashes, Scribonius also gives treatments for the relief of toothache consisting of a variety of herbal rinses:

1. The root of parieta cooked in wine
2. Pellitory and cypress berries cooked in water
3. Hyoscyamus root or seed, wrapped in cloth and boiled in water
4. Purslane, chewed, and its juice held in the mouth
5. The lukewarm juice of solanum mixed with lignite

Besides the treatments described above which were provided by literary sources, archaeological research has discovered evidence for the innovative manufacture and use of replacement teeth. The Etruscan origins of gold dental prosthetics from the middle of the seventh century BC are well recognised. These flat gold bands were fashioned to hold a tooth, or a number of teeth, in place. About twenty such items have been documented, of which nine are extant. Recent research using odontometrics, combined with archaeological data, suggests that the appliances were used only by women.[26] It is implied that high-status Etruscan women deliberately had their teeth removed in order for them to be attached to a gold band. Tooth-loss was an accepted part of ageing in the ancient world and deliberate tooth removal is known from many areas in antiquity, besides Italy. It is also known in the modern world. The decline of Etruscan culture, including the use of the Etruscan language, in the face of dominance from Rome, in addition to changing fashions over the years, partly explains why these appliances have disappeared. There is no known archaeological evidence for the continuation of these objects into the Roman period, although this does not entirely preclude their possible manufacture and use at this time.

An item of related interest was found at the Roman cemeteries at Kelvedon, in Essex.[27] The only Roman burial there about which we possess specific information comprised a plain monolithic coffin and lid of oolite limestone containing 'a lady with a false tooth of pebble buried in plaster'. The contents of the coffin were not kept, and there were no grave-goods. However, from a Gallo-Roman necropolis at Chatambre (Essonne, France) a find of an even more exciting nature has been reported; this is no less than the perfect replica of a human tooth, the wrought-iron dental implant of a right second upper premolar,[28] dating from the first or second century AD. The fit of the implant within the tooth socket is reportedly excellent, plus there is complete ante-mortem integration of the bone with the metal object. The fabrication of the detailed replica of a human tooth successfully implanted into the jaw is as amazing and deserving of admiration, as are the survival rates of those who underwent the surgical operation of trephination (see below).

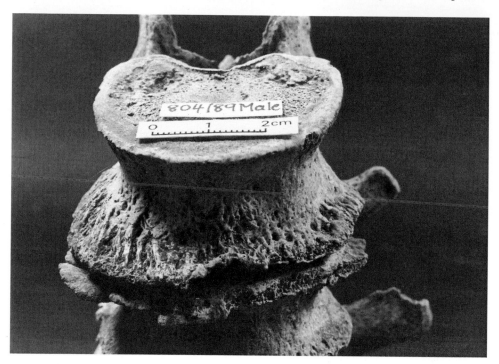

84 Part of the lumbar spine of a male skeleton excavated at Sherston; prominent osteophytes are present on the vertebral bodies. These are associated with heavy manual labour, especially lifting and carrying over a long period of time

Dr Calvin Wells' views, expressed in 1964 before scientific procedures were as fully developed as they are now, continue to be valid despite the emergence of new diseases, such as AIDS and the human form of BSE. His text remains as true today as then; the precepts expressed have never been told more clearly:

> The pattern of disease or injury that affects any group of people is never a matter of chance. It is invariably the expression of stresses and strains to which they were exposed, a response to everything in their environment and behaviour. It reflects their genetic inheritance (which is their internal environment), the climate in which they lived, the soil that gave them sustenance and the animals or plants that shared their homeland. It is influenced by their daily occupations, their habits of diet, their choice of dwelling and clothes, their social structure, even their folklore and mythology. This realisation that 'Man is a whole with his environment', though at least as old as Galen, is still a neglected precept despite the fact that it underlies the study of disease, in ancient peoples no less than in the living... for the more intimate knowledge of how people have responded to the aggression of their environment pathology is a surer guide.[29] (*84*).

PALAEOPATHOLOGY AND ROMAN BODIES — POMPEII

In AD 79 the eruption of Vesuvius destroyed several Campanian towns and villas, including Pompeii and Herculaneum. The layer of thick volcanic ash resulted in the preservation, among other artefacts, of gardens, buildings, wall-paintings, sculpture and the skeletal remains of victims. All these categories of evidence have been scrutinised in the quest to illuminate the lives of the people of Pompeii. Such lacunae can now be filled out more faithfully by a careful study of their bones. The examination of recently found skeletons, in the light of new advances in palaeopathology, provides a rare insight into the life and health of the people of Pompeii and Herculaneum in the first century AD.[30]

The original excavation of the town began in 1748. The main aim of the early excavators was finding treasure. Skeletons were merely a grim reminder of the ever-present, smouldering presence of the volcanic mountain. Any bones that were retained were used to create macabre displays for the enjoyment of visiting worthies. Initially, before ever bone-analysis was known, it had long been assumed that the skeletons found at Pompeii belonged to the elderly and the infirm and the women and children, who would have been unable to move fast enough to escape the suffocating volcanic fall-out. However, due to recent discoveries of skeletons within the layer of pumice and fine ash, it became possible to challenge this assumption. Many of the skeletons were disarticulated and partial and the lack of complete skeletons was a handicap to research. A further difficulty encountered by the researcher[31] was the lack of access to laboratory facilities and X-ray equipment. Therefore, only hands-on methods, such as those described above, could be used. Despite all these difficulties, work continued and some valuable findings were made. The purpose of the investigation was to discover whether the people who remained at Pompeii, and who subsequently suffered the full and fatal onslaught of the eruption, did so through choice or through dire necessity. Was their escape from all the horrors of it prevented by physical limitations, and if so what form did these take?

All volcanic eruptions are different and analogy must be used with caution. However, after studying the volcanology of Vesuvius by using for a model the similar, two-phase eruption of Mount St Helens in Washington in 1984, and also by scrutinising the skeletal remains for disease or injury, the researcher decided that escape would have been physically possible for most inhabitants of the city. Moreover, even if the victims were elderly or infirm, there would have been enough time for the escape to have occurred during the eighteen-hour pumice and ash fall-out. However, this was followed by fast-travelling hot-gas avalanches and at this stage little free oxygen would have been available. All this was accompanied by a turbulent, highly toxic gas content in the atmosphere, at which stage escape would have been impossible. The experience at Pompeii would have been terrifying, with overall darkness and a constant hail of small pumice stones raining on the victims for hours and hours, so that all levels of the remaining community would have been equally affected. It was suggested by the researcher that this group of people probably, though fatally, decided to wait out the eruption.

The adult skeletal material at Pompeii showed no significant age or sex bias. Children were not well represented, but this was thought to be due to the small bones being either not recognised, or else lost. Conversely, perhaps, the children escaped. The degree of injury found in the skeletons was small. However, healed fractures in long bones showed misalignment, and a healed, depressed skull-fracture was also seen. Judging by the position of the latter fracture, brain damage would most certainly have resulted from this injury. With regard to joint-disease, it was found to be difficult to separate bony changes as a result of trauma from age-related diseases, because the whole skeleton is required for such a differential diagnosis. However, two age-related diseases were found and these are now described.

The first is diffuse ideopathic hyperostosis (Forestier's disease), more commonly known as 'DISH', which mainly affects the spinal column. The cause is unknown but it is often associated with diabetes and obesity. The spine becomes completely fused, particularly in the thoracic region. Extremely large bone cells, or osteophytes, are produced, which flow like candlewax along the anterior longitudinal ligament. It is especially interesting to find this at Pompeii as it is more often associated with the elderly inhabitants of medieval monastic cemeteries. DISH is not particularly debilitating and is most often only diagnosed post-mortem.

Hyperostosis frontalis interna was another sub-clinical condition found at Pompeii. This is a disorder which may have caused headache in middle-aged, post-menopausal females. It is characterised by a bilateral, symmetrical thickening of the endocranial surface of the frontal bone of the skull and may begin after a pregnancy. HFI was assumed to be rare in antiquity because of the shorter life-span at that time. It is seldom reported in the archaeological literature. Out of the 360 skulls examined at Pompeii, changes consistent with HFI were present in forty-three individuals. The researcher suggests that this indicates a life-span at Pompeii comparable to that of today.

In addition to an insight into the terrifying experience of a particular volcanic eruption, we are given a snap-shot of the health and longevity of the population of Pompeii, as well as of possible medical intervention. Although fractures were set in the Roman period, the three misaligned fractures found at Pompeii appear not to have been treated. However, unequivocal surgical intervention was seen in two cases of trephination. Judged by the degree of healing that had taken place, both operations appeared to have been performed before death, with proven survival of the patient. One of them may have been performed to alleviate the headache of the individual with HFI, on whom the surgery had been performed. The operation, though successful, would not have helped the headache, however, as this condition is of hormonal origin.

Many sets of surgical instruments were discovered at both Pompeii and Herculaneum, and several physicians are known to have practised in these towns. However this is not attested in the skeletal evidence and it is concluded that these individuals did not have access to doctors for financial, social or other reasons – archaeologists are not privy to the very private and personal minutiae of people's lives. The researcher concluded that the individuals who were caught in the volcanic fall-out were not the most elderly and infirm members of their society, but people who, for reasons we cannot know, decided to sit it out and wait.

HERCULANEUM

As enquiry continues into the skeletal reports, it is clear that the study of human skeletal material has an immediacy that is not as readily available to other studies in antiquity, except, perhaps, for that of epigraphy. Human remains bring us face to face with individuals. This is most sensibly apparent in the example of a young woman from Herculaneum.[32] Here, the accidental discovery, in the spring of 1982, of a large number of skeletons on the beach front and others in a nearby boat-house, changed the interpretation of history. Previously, since few skeletons had been found at Herculaneum, scholars had believed that almost all the people left town before the eruption of Vesuvius on 24 August, AD 79. However, as a result of recent findings, we are fortunate in being able to view the situation differently. Due to their long-term burial under 20m of volcanic material, the newly-discovered skeletons were held in an unchanging temperature for 1,900 years and, when found, were in good condition.

Several of the skeletons are of particular interest; two of them will be discussed. The first is a young woman known as 'Erc 52'. Based on her epiphyses, the age of 'Erc 52' was estimated at about twenty-six years. Small bones found within the pelvic area demonstrated that she was pregnant with a foetus of about seven months when the catastrophe occurred, the age of the foetus being based on the length of the long bones. Although 'Erc 52' was shorter than the population mean, this was found, after examination of her bones and teeth, not to have been caused by poor nutrition or ill-health, but to some other factor, such as family characteristics. Her small musculature was probably due to her genetic inheritance in combination with a fairly easy and comfortable way of life. A touching detail is that in the rush to escape the lava-flow by boat, she fell and the house or boat-house key that she was carrying became lodged in her hair, causing the formation of iron-rust on her scalp. When carefully examined, some of her long, blond hair was found to have been preserved in the rust. This is a primary, if poignant, example of the preservation of organic material by contact with metal corrosion products. The organic material is, of course, a source of DNA.

Another especially interesting case from Herculaneum is that of a child, 'Erc 8'. Judging from the iliac crest, the skeleton was most probably that of a female, and based on the stage of her tooth development, she was about seven years old. The lengths of her long bones show her to be of small stature, now judged to be normal for that population. The most interesting feature was a healed greenstick fracture of the distal shaft of the right forearm of both radius and ulna. The shaft of these bones was markedly swollen when compared with the bones of the left arm, and the fractured radius was bent posteriorly in its displacement. The child probably fell from a height onto the outstretched arm and would have experienced great pain for several weeks as a result of the untreated fracture.

SKELETAL EVIDENCE FOR TREPHINATION

It is often stated that trepanation, or the surgical removal of a portion of the skull, is the earliest surgical operation to have been performed, but this is most unlikely to be true. What is true, however, is that this particular surgical intervention has left clear skeletal evidence that it was, indeed, practised in antiquity. Evidence for the procedure is recognised from the Mesolithic and Neolithic periods until later times. A ritual or magical component cannot be ruled out, particularly in Iron-Age Britain, where many examples are seen. It seems that for ancient societies the soul was supposed to reside in the head. Evil spirits, to which headache, bad dreams or nightmares were attributed, could be 'let out' by the extraction of roundels of bone from the cranium; these objects were often much prized for use as amulets.

Two crown trephines of the kind described by Celsus were found with a set of finely-wrought instruments excavated from a late first-century tomb at Bingen-am-Rhein, near Mainz, in Germany.[33] This type of surgical tool was widely used in the Roman period. It could well have been used at York where, in the nineteenth century, a Romano-British site was under excavation in preparation for the construction of the railway.[34] A case of trephination was found here and, judging from the evidence of the cranial morphology and the teeth, it was decided that the skeleton was that of an adult female. The serration of the hole made by the surgeon in the temporal bone did not completely sever the disc of bone away from the skull, but possibly this was deliberate; the operation carried out thus far would have relieved intra-cranial pressure and may have been considered sufficient for the relief of 'pains in the head'. Moreover, the actual method employed is not in doubt; the pronounced circular 'boring' is unlikely to have been produced by any other tool than that circular modiolus.[35] There are no signs of healing or inflammation of the surrounding bone, so it is assumed that the patient did not survive the ordeal.

Although trephined skulls in the Roman period are not numerous, it is possible to mention a few examples. The skull found at Cirencester is of particular interest;[36] inhumation 305 was a male who had received a severe gash across his right parietal bone. In addition to incising the bone, the blow had severely fractured the skull so that a triangular area had parted from it and was depressed inwards. In life it would have caused damage to the meninges with possible neurological impairment. An eliptical opening with smoothly bevelled sides was also found in the frontal bone; this appeared to be a trephination. It was probably performed in an attempt to relieve the symptoms caused by the trauma. Despite the severity of the injury, the subsequent surgery seems to have been successful, and the wound eventually healed well.

A trephined skull found at the Roman cemetery in Newarke Street, Leicester in 1993/4, testifies to the skill of such an operator as we have seen working at Cirencester.[37] The left parietal bone of the male skeleton (inhumation 424) (*85* and *86*) showed a healed depressed fracture which resembled a 'saucer-shaped hollow'; there was also a neat circular hole, with flat, slightly bevelled sides on the left-hand side of the frontal bone. This showed no

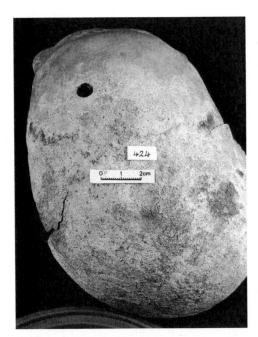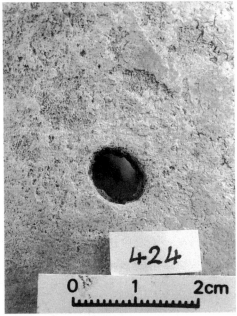

85 Left a) The skull vault of a male skeleton from Newarke Street, Leicester. A trephined opening can be seen in the frontal bone. An indentation in the midline posteriorly shows a well-healed depressed fracture; *Right* b) Close up view of the trephination. There is no evidence of healing, indicating that the patient did not survive the surgery

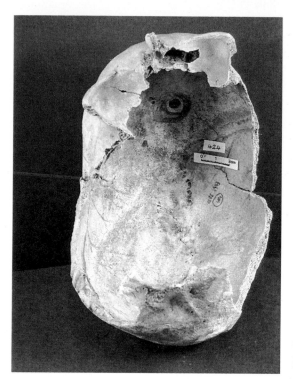

86 Interior view of the skull of the male patient from Newarke Street. A neat round trephined opening can be seen in the frontal bone, surrounded by post-mortem deposits of salts from the burial environment

signs of healing around its edges, thus demonstrating that it was made at, or shortly before, the man's death. The technique used was probably that of the modiolus as described by Celsus and the operation was most likely to have been an attempt to treat symptoms arising from the earlier depressed fracture; an attempt, perhaps, to relieve a headache. The author of the skeletal report, Dr Wakely, comments as follows: 'the evidence for the practice of trepanation points to the presence there of a surgeon capable of undertaking such a heroic procedure. Whether this person was a resident of Leicester, or an itinerant specialist as existed in other fields of medicine in the Roman Empire, cannot be determined. The skill of the operator and the courage of the patient both deserve our admiration.'[38] Unfortunately, however, this patient did not survive the operation.

In the two cases of trephination encountered at Pompeii, above, and those more recently discussed, it has been seen that the procedure is most usually suspected to have been employed to treat 'pains in the head', or headache. This was a condition considered by Pliny, together with bladder-stone and stomach ailments, to cause the sharpest agony. He writes, *Nat. Hist.* 25.7.24, 'these are the only diseases that are responsible for suicides'. In view of what is known of other possibilities for suicide, both in ancient and in modern times, this might seem to be a somewhat sweeping or naïve comment. But we need to think historically and to realise that several diseases, some unknown today due to improvements in medical practices, were much feared in the ancient world and that headache in particular was feared because it would have been experienced as an early symptom of any one of them. No knowledge of bacteriology meant, of course, no availability of antibiotics, and an agonising and protracted death was often inevitable and also to be dreaded. In modern times, although sometimes used in excess, or inappropriately, chemotherapy can be lifesaving. If such diseases as the frequent plagues, malarias, puerperal fevers and septicaemia are kept in mind – or, indeed, other severe illnesses, any of which could have given rise to such symptoms as headache, high fevers or stomach pain – it becomes clear that these are conditions from which, without recourse to effective treatment, people seldom had hope of recovery. Thus, fear of prolonged suffering ending in death would have been very great. In such circumstances an easier and planned death by suicide may have been a longed-for alternative. It is from this perspective that the comment of Pliny should be considered.

Intense fear would also have been suffered by those who willingly underwent the operation of trephination. The patient would most probably have needed to be forcibly restrained. Pain relief may have been obtained by the administration of drugs such as alcohol, opium, henbane or mandrake. Possibly, these were included in the many different and arcane theriacs that were used in antiquity. This would have been a hit-or-miss affair and great courage and trust would have been required on the part of both the patient and the operator. The scene itself is difficult to imagine, imbued as we are with modern science, medical expertise and comfort and cleanliness. Nevertheless, it has been demonstrated above that there were surprising successes in the field of medicine in antiquity and the courage and skills demonstrated by physicians in this early time of medical enquiry and discovery are fully deserving of our admiration.

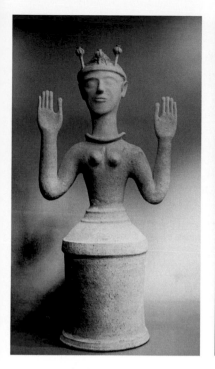
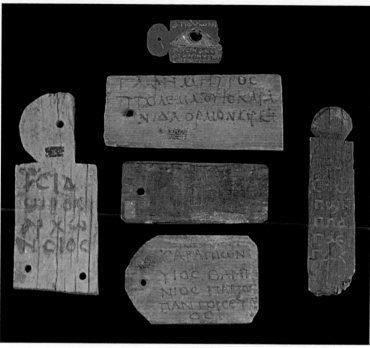

1 Left The Gazi goddess, a late Minoan figurine; *2 Right* Top object is a greenish-grey fragmentary schist apotropaic eye with Greek inscription *c.*second century AD, with an inlaid white glass eye, blue glass pupil, bronze surround, and an invocation to 'golden Apollo, grace on behalf of a daughter'. *Courtesy Emma Sully, Christie's*

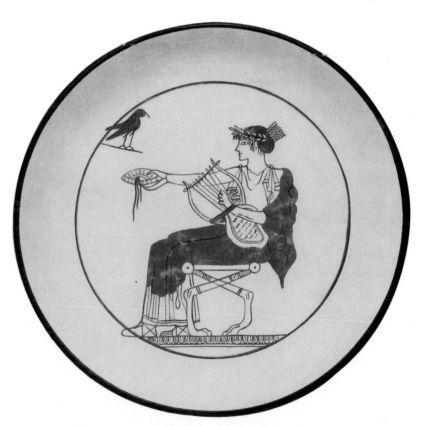

3 Apollo pours a libation. Copy of a white kylix, fifth century BC

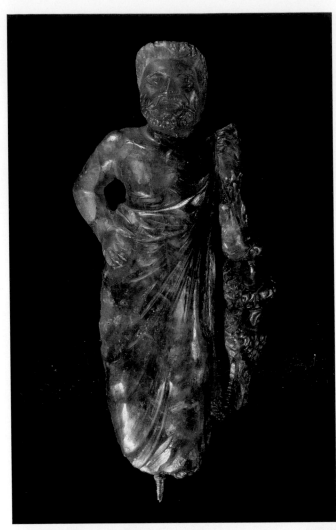

4 *Left* Fluorite figurine of Asklepius (Henig 1990, no.181). *Content Family Collection, by permission of Philippa Content*

5 *Below left* Onyx cameo in gold pendant showing Asclepius, Hygea and Telesphorus (Henig and Vickers 1993, 33, fig. 2.6). *Content Family Collection, by permission of Philippa Content*

6 *Below right* Onyx cameo of three layers, white on dark brown, bluish-white, black showing Asklepius, Hygea and Telesphorus (Henig 1990, no.88). *Content Family Collection, by permission of Philippa Content*

Opposite page:
7 *Above* A second- or third-century Roman mosaic showing the arrival at Cos of the god Asklepius, disembarking from a boat and being welcomed by a wayfarer with a gesture of surprise and adoration. Hippocrates sits on a raised stone, symbolising the island of his birth; he is plainly recognisable by his posture as a teacher. *Bulletino D'Arte, 35, 1950*

8 *Below left* Statue of Hygea from Cos Museum

9 *Below right* A statue of Hippocrates from Cos

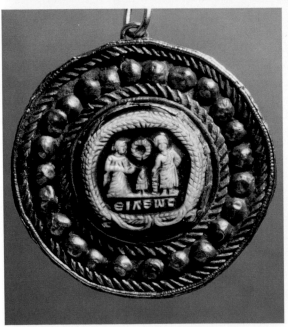

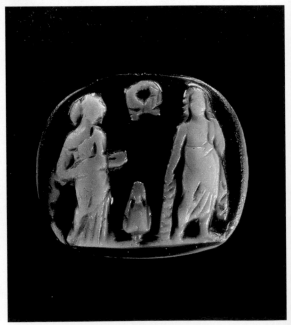

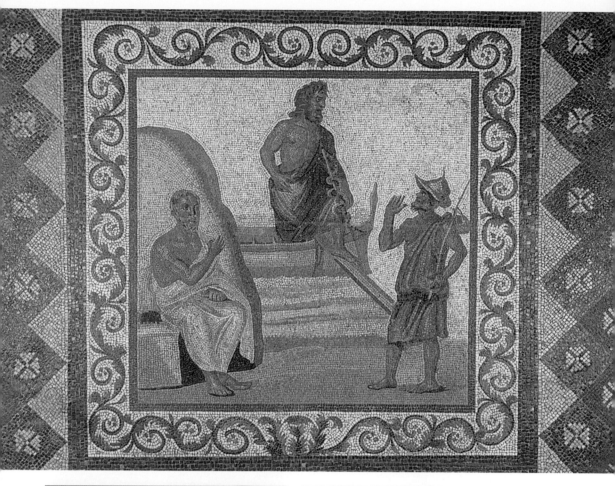

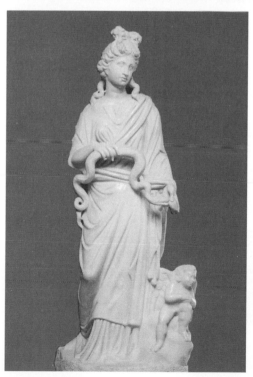

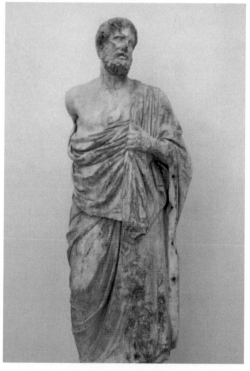

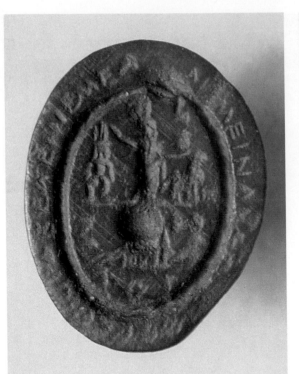
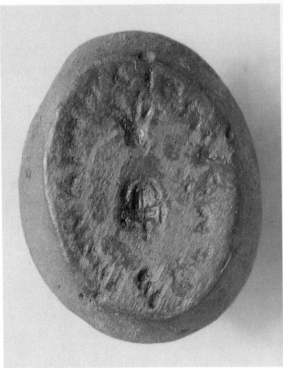

10 Double-sided haematite amulet from Welwyn, *RIB* 2423.1. *Institute of Archaeology, Oxford*

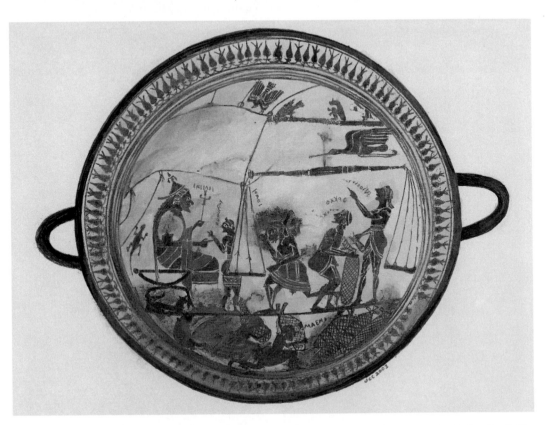

11 King Arkesilas (possibly) supervising the weighing of silphium. Painting after a Laconian kylix, first half of the sixth century BC. *Paris Bibliothèque Nationale*

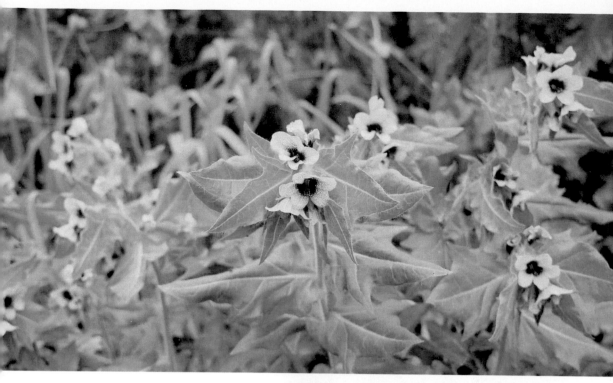

12 *Above* Henbane, *Hyoscamus niger*

13 *Datura stramonium*
Below a) the flower
Right b) in the courtyard of
Wolfson College, Oxford

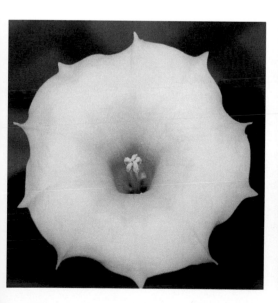

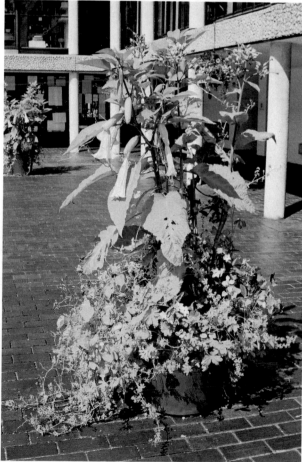

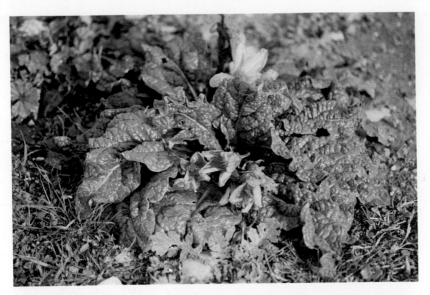

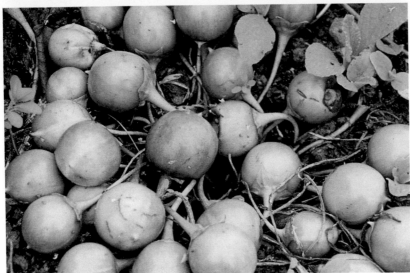

14 *Above left* a) Flower of the mandrake growing in Tunisia; *Left* b) *Mandragora officianarum* at Chelsea Physic Garden

15 *Below Atropa belladonna* growing in the Oxford Botanical Gardens

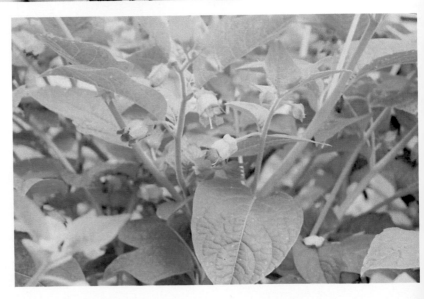

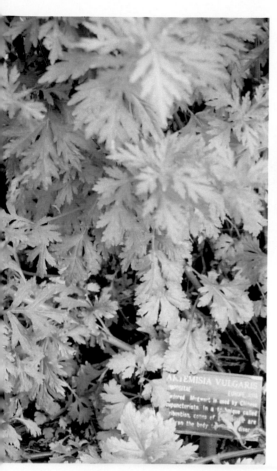

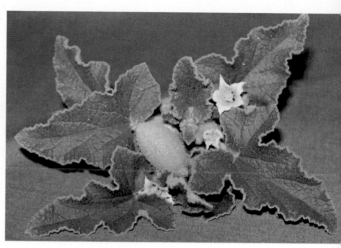

16 Left Artemisia vulgaris in the Chelsea Physic Garden

17 Above Echallium elaterium (squirting cucumber) growing at Mycenae; 'There is a wild cucumber much smaller than the cultivated kind. From it is made the drug called *elaterium*', Pliny, *Nat. Hist.* 20.2. It is a cure-all; among other maladies it is useful for painful joints and sinusitis

18 Below Valeriana officinalis in the Chelsea Physic Garden

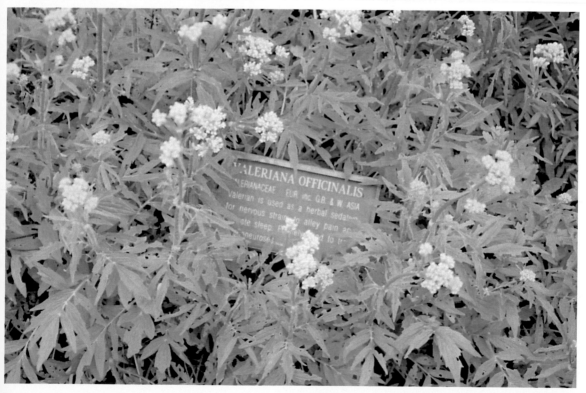

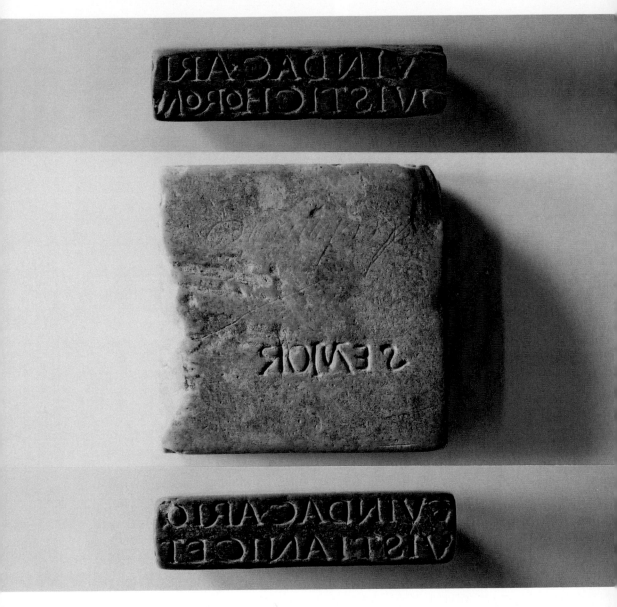

19 The collyrium stamp of Titus Vindacius Ariovistus from Kenchester (*RIB* 2446.3), showing two of the inscriptions, cut in retrograde; on the sides of the tablet which are not illustrated is inscribed (a) 'Titus Vindacius Ar|iovistus' nard-oil salve', (b) 'Titus Vindacius Ari|ovistus' green salve' and (c) 'Titus Vindacius Ario|vistus' infallible salve'. *Courtesy of the British Museum*

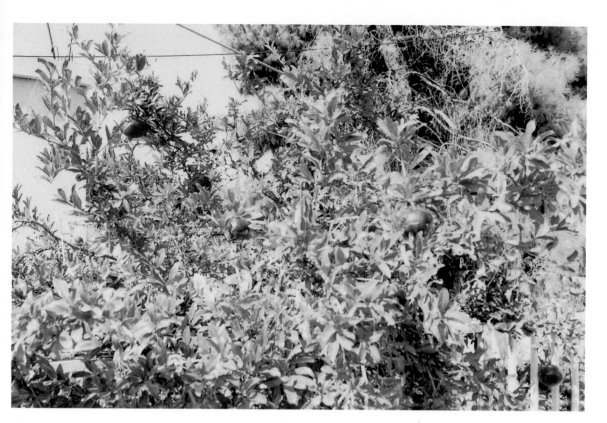

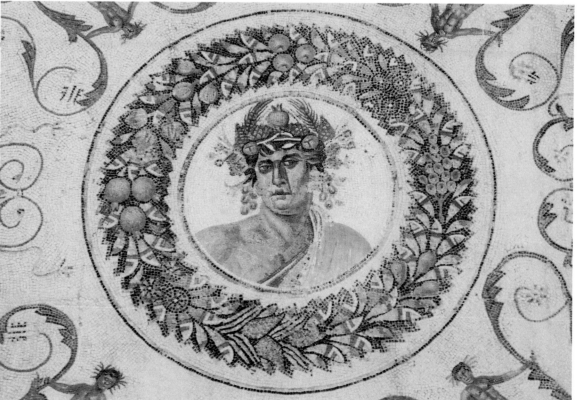

20 Above a) A pomegranate tree growing in Corinth; *Below* b) Pomegranates also featured plentifully in the frieze surrounding the bust of Bacchus on a North African mosaic

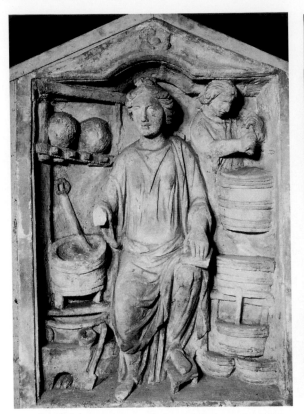
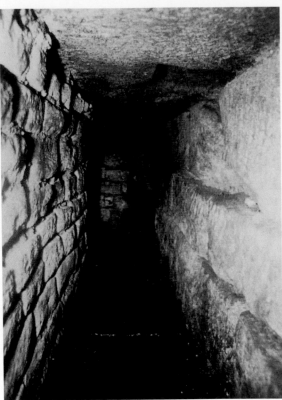

21 Above left A Roman relief supposed to be showing soap and salve making. An assistant appears to grind ingredients using a pestle and mortar; the products could have been simmered in a cauldron over a furnace, left, and stored in vats, right; *22 Above right* Part of a Roman sewer system beneath the legionary fortress at York

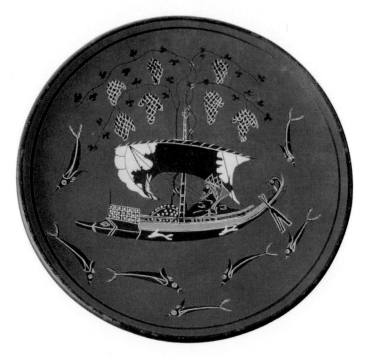

23 Dionysus brings the grape to Europe; a copy of the plate of Exekias made in the mid-sixth century BC, Munich

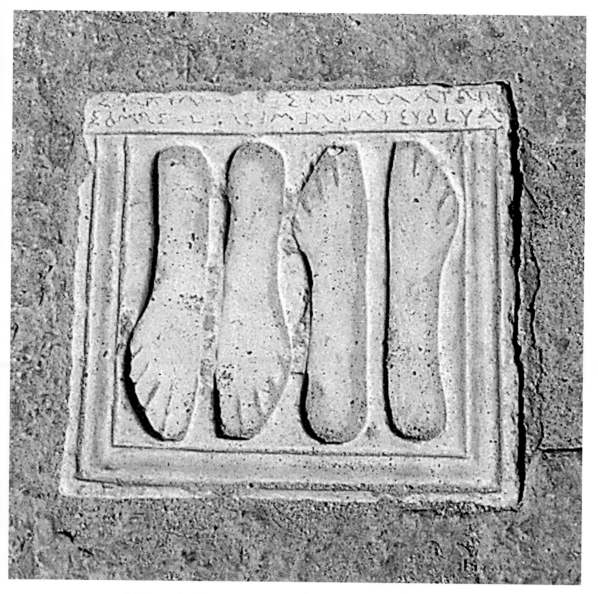

24 Votive feet from Italica, dedicated to the goddess Nemesis-Caelestis

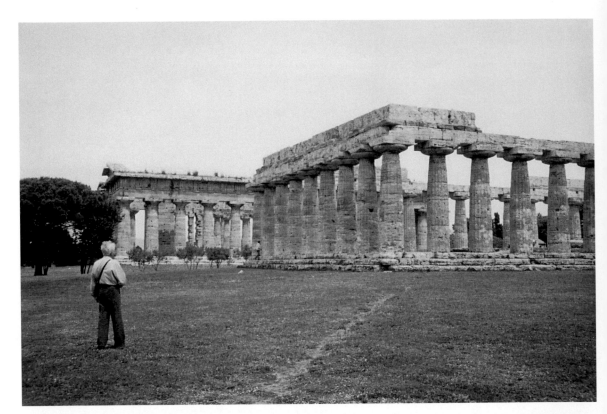

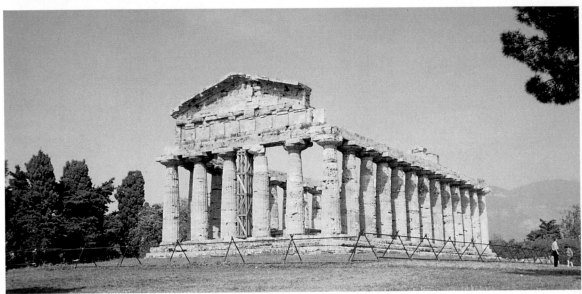

25 Paestum: the Doric temples. *Above* Temple of Hera I ('Basilica'), mid-sixth century and Temple of Hera II, mid-fifth century. *Below* Temple of Athena, late sixth century

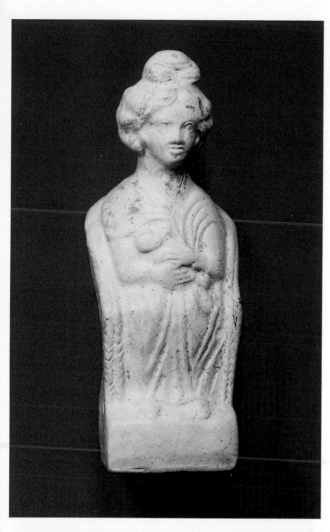

26 *Left* Pipeclay figurine of a mother goddess suckling an infant. From Welwyn, England, second century AD

27 *Below* Copy of a bronze hound of Nodens from Lydney, Gloucestershire

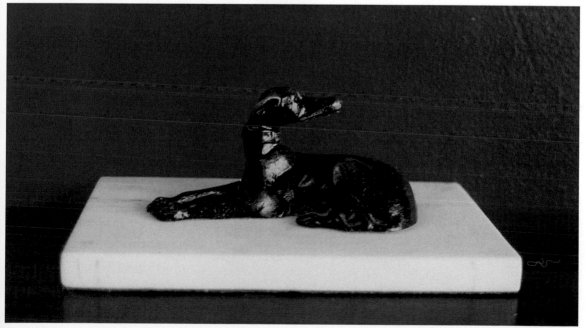

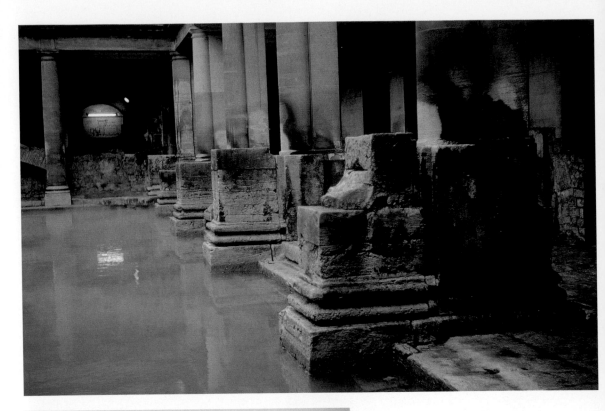

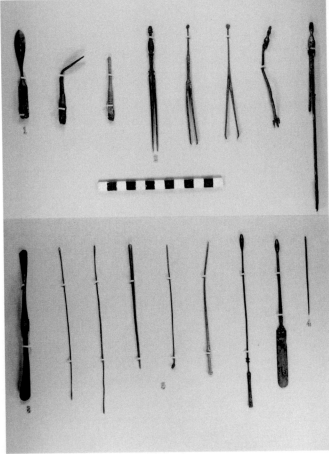

28 *Above* The Great Bath at Bath. In Roman times the bath was enclosed

29 *Left* A variety of surgical instruments in the Romano-British collection of the British Museum: (1) Three scalpel handles; the iron blades have corroded away; (2) Five spring forceps; the one with the pointed jaws could have been used in fine surgery, the two with inturned smooth jaws were dissecting tools, the fifth example was converted in antiquity into a three-pronged fork; (3) Iron curette, combining a spatulate lever and a sharp-rimmed scoop probably for work in bone surgery; (4) Iron needle; (5) Seven bronze probes, used in exploratory work on wounds, sinuses etc.; the finest was a double-ended probe, *diprene*

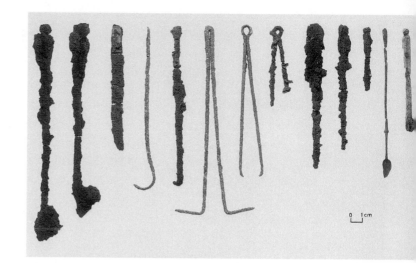

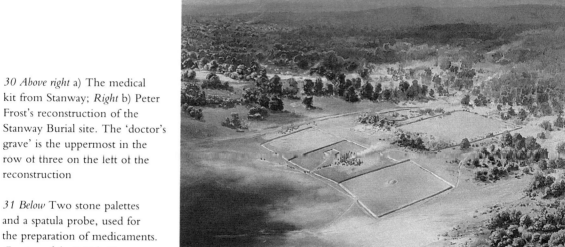

30 *Above right* a) The medical kit from Stanway; *Right* b) Peter Frost's reconstruction of the Stanway Burial site. The 'doctor's grave' is the uppermost in the row of three on the left of the reconstruction

31 *Below* Two stone palettes and a spatula probe, used for the preparation of medicaments. *Courtesy of the British Museum*

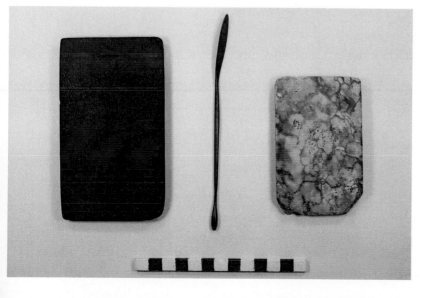

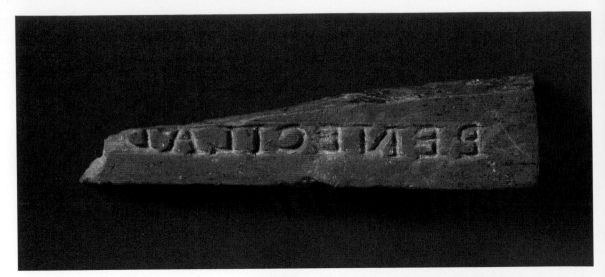

32 *Above* The collyrium stamp from the
macellum site at Wroxeter. The inscription
reads *'penecilai'*, the salve of Lucillianus for
lippitudo. Found in 1981 in a third or early
fourth century pit.

33 *Right* Base of a samian cup with
impressions of a collyrium stamp. It reads
'Lucius Iulius Senex's saffron salve for
granulation of the eyelids'

34 *Below right* Romano-British collyrium
stamps in the British Museum

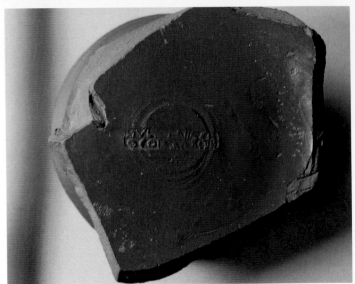

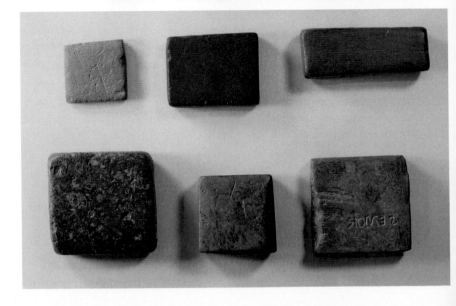

— 8 —

PHYSICIANS AND HEALERS
IN THE ROMAN WORLD

I would require Honesty in every Physician, that he be not over careless or covetous, Harpylike to make a prey of his patient, or, as an hungry Chirurgeon, often produce and wire-draw his cure, so long as there is any hope of pay. Many of them, to get a fee, will give physic to everyone that comes, when there is no cause, thus, as it often falleth out, stirring up a silent disease, and making a strong body weak.

Robert Burton, 1577-1650, *The Anatomy of Melancholy*

This affectionate satire on the vagaries of physicians may belong to another era, but its application to the medical practices of antiquity is strikingly apt. Moreover, it is a reminder that the doctors of antiquity who have come down to us, either in their own writings or in the texts of later recorders, and who are described below, are mainly those of good reputation. Another 'crowd of physicians' (to quote from Pliny, *Nat. Hist.* 29.5.11) was also around, many of whom remain unknown. What is known, however, is that Oribasius (AD 325-97), physician to the Emperor Julian, was concerned about the state of medicine at this later period of the Roman Empire for he complained about the numbers of inept doctors and the lack of useful handbooks. Several doctors in this period are known to us by name but, regretfully, in most cases, only small fragments of their works survive. Such writings as have come down to us are merely the accidental survivors of time. They form only a small portion of the quantity of texts that would have been available in antiquity.

In writing here of Roman doctors and Roman medicine, reference is made to the Graeco-Roman medicine of the late Roman Republic and Empire. Although an extensive geographical area is encompassed in the survey, this should not be taken to indicate that ways of healing were identical throughout the Empire. In rural areas, particular local customs and prejudices prevailed. For

193

most of the population, however, medical treatment would have consisted of agrarian self-help and medico-magical remedies. Suppliers of drugs and practitioners of healing were available in the towns, for it was with city-life and Hellenisation that Greek medicine arrived in Italy and was further disseminated through the western provinces. The divisions, so fiercely censured by Cato and Pliny, although in part due to cultural factors, were probably less between Greek and Roman than between urban and non-urban environments,[1] or, to be more specific, they were between rustic medicine and that of the big city.

THE MEDICAE, THE MEDICI AND THE PATIENTS

Although in ancient Greece women remained in the home and a few in wealthy families received education there, they were not permitted to follow a profession and would certainly not have been able to become doctors.[2] In the Roman Empire, however, women were treated differently. Roman women were not restricted to a domestic life. They were able to take part in some of the same activities as men. The Vindolanda letters[3] indicate that women were literate. A Roman wife was able to divorce her husband and furthermore, if necessary, she could retain custody of the children. Many professions, including medicine, were open to both sexes. Soranus' midwife is always referred to as 'she', but male physicians could also attend women patients; a good example is, of course, Soranus himself. Some women doctors, *medicae*, were well thought of and were commemorated in funerary inscriptions. An inscription from Spain (*CIL* 11 492 = *ILS* 7802) tells of Iulius Saturnina of Merida. It was set up by her husband to 'an incomparable wife, the best physician, a most virtuous woman'.[4] Another inscription found on a relief from second-century AD Ostia cites Scribonia Attica, a midwife whose husband, M. Ulpius Amerimnus, was a doctor and surgeon.[5]

Professional doctors in Italy were normally immigrants. Claudius Agathemerus, whose funerary monument is displayed in the Ashmolean Museum, came from Sparta (*87*). Translated,[6] the inscription reads:

> Claudius Agathemerus a doctor, I lie here
> Knowledgeable in swift remedies for all kinds of illness
> I have set up this common memorial for myself and my wife Myrtale
> We are together with the blessed in Eleusis.

Archagathus, the 'wound doctor' (*vulnerarius medicus*), whether or not he was the first Greek doctor to set up practice at Rome in 219 BC, as claimed by Pliny (*Nat. Hist.* 29.6.12), was the first to be employed by the Roman state. This was a considerable step towards the official sanctioning of a public health service. Although the authorities, both civil and imperial, were interested in

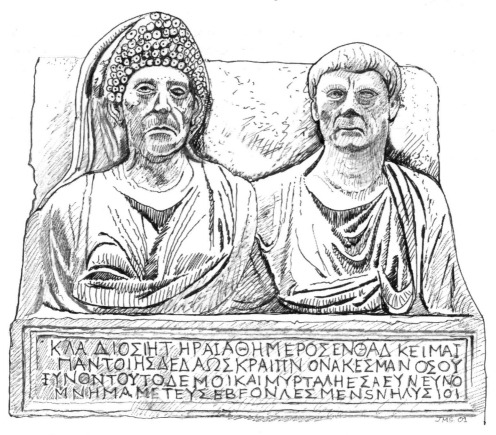

87 Tombstone found in Rome of the Spartan doctor Claudius Agathemerus and his wife

defining who could be a 'doctor', there were no official medical examinations or degrees leading to qualifications. The success of a physician and the scale of his income depended upon his reputation. For this reason terminally ill patients or uncertain cases were not treated.

On the authority of Pliny (*Nat. Hist.* 29), the appointment of Archagathus in 219 BC ended in disaster when, following his savage use of the knife and cautery, he and all physicians became objects of loathing. It was not until the reign of Julius Caesar, some one-and-a-half centuries later, that the state intervened again in public health. Around the year 40 BC, according to Suetonius, 'Julius Caesar granted the citizenship to all medical practitioners resident in Rome, thus inducing them to remain … and tempting others to follow suit', (Suet. *Jul.* 42).

With citizenship came exemption from paying certain taxes. One reason for such concessions could have been to encourage more doctors to work in Rome, where their numbers may have been seriously depleted by military service. Such a move on the part of the state indicates that physicians were not only necessary but were also much valued.[7] Jackson suggests that Caesar's appreciation of doctors is shown in his linking them with teachers of the liberal arts. Under Hadrian their privileges were the same as those accorded to firemen and transport workers, perhaps an acknowledgement of their practical skills. Caesar's tax exemptions for doctors in Rome soon applied to physicians throughout the empire. In addition, they were excused from having soldiers billeted on them.[8] The same privileges were continued by subsequent rulers. However, in AD 150, Emperor Antoninus Pius restricted the number of 'approved' doctors to a maximum of five, seven or ten according to the size and status of their towns.

The decision over who qualified for tax concessions was not made by medical personnel but by magistrates or other non-medical officers of the state. It is possible that ulterior motives, such as the need for access to medical assistance (perhaps touching on legal services connected with violent death or injury), influenced their judgements. However, such methods could have been no guarantee of medical competence and several tales of cobblers or gladiators becoming doctors overnight are found in the literary sources.[9] This meant, of course, that the assessment of medical competence rested in public opinion, which is easily swayed, or silenced, and is therefore seldom a reliable indicator. Even in modern Britain, in a recent infamous case, a doctor managed to murder many scores of his patients and to remain undetected for a long time.

Although medical books were not easily obtainable, Celsus' *De Medicina* was available to buy for those who could read and were wealthy enough to be able to purchase books. Works of other writers, such as Scribonius Largus (*c.*AD 1–50), Pliny (*c.*AD 23–79) and Pedanius Dioscorides (*c.*AD 40–90) may also have been accessible. Doctors who were resident in imperial palaces, for example Galen who lived at the courts of emperors – Marcus Aurelius, his son Commodus, and Septimius Severus – would have had easier access to both medical literature and the best drugs and equipment. Some teachers of medicine allowed their lectures to be written down and circulated. Public anatomy displays, such as the dissections performed on animals, both dead and alive, given by Galen, took place. Lectures were also given in the town gymnasium. Medical education was not, however, formalised, although teachers attracted groups of followers. Pupils could also accompany doctors on their rounds, sometimes as apprentices. The probable existence of hospitals may be inferred from the comment of Celsus, *De Med. Prooemium* 65, where he refers to 'those who take charge of large hospitals'. However, no other information, whether archaeological or literary, is known for the presence of civilian hospitals until late antiquity.

In the event of accident or illness, many people, especially the poor, would have had to rely on self-help or support within the family. For the wealthy there were other options: people could be treated in their own homes by resident or visiting physicians. 'Public' physicians would have had premises in the towns, either in their homes or in a *taberna medica*, such as might have been found in a side street among other shops occupied by tradespeople of all sorts. Wherever doctors' premises are known, it is because their identity has been confirmed by finds of medical instruments or equipment.

The expansion of Roman territory in the second century BC brought great wealth to the Empire. This led to profound changes in economic and social life in all Italy. Industry and commerce intensified and slavery increased, both on the land and in the household. *Luxuria* was greatly enjoyed and Greek influence was seen to be present in many aspects of daily life, for example, in art and architecture, literature and religion. Greek ways of living, together with their styles of dress and person, were much admired, studied and followed. In contrast to his writings, in which he complained about Greeks and their medicine, Cato spent his last years learning their language. Another effect to follow from the general prosperity was the rich pickings available to innovative and charming *medici*.

The following discussion is an elucidation continued from pp.49-50. In the late second century BC,[10] at the time when Asclepiades of Bithynia was making a brilliant success of medical practice at Rome, the most well-known physicians could be divided into two main groups, Dogmatists (also known as Rationalists) and Empiricists. Although there were differences between individuals, the situation was essentially as follows: Dogmatists insisted on obtaining knowledge of the hidden causes of disease. They based medicine on theory, even to the extent of allowing academic reasoning to go beyond sober science. They used observation and speculation in varying degrees, to make conclusions about the composition of the human body, the nature of health and disease and the processes of life itself. Empiricists, however, embraced an opposite viewpoint. Rejecting enquiry into hidden causes, they claimed that dissection revealed nothing about the living and that it merely provided information about the dead. In the view of Empiricists, nature itself was incomprehensible. They prefered to rely on their own experience and the accumulated experience from the past. In the first century AD, in opposition to these extreme positions, Methodism arose. Themison of Laodicia, *fl. c.*70 BC, who had been a pupil of Asclepiades, gave the initial impetus to this movement.

Methodists reacted against and rejected both groups. Methodist scepticism was less radical than that of the Empiricists. They left open the possibility of revisions on the basis of new observations. For them, Empiricism was too extreme. On the other hand, Dogmatic science, in their view, was no more than an intellectual exercise, of no use whatsoever to the practice of medicine. Methodists made their own broad classifications of disease based on what they could see to be the case. Their focus of interest was the individual patient and their motivation was built on therapeutic principles. Rejecting the Hippocratic theory of the four humours, Methodist physicians constructed a physiology founded on the theory of atoms. In this theory the proper arrangement of atoms and their immediate pores produced good health. Obstruction or looseness in the atoms led to diseases which were classified as acute or chronic, requiring either dietetic or pharmacological treatment, or surgery. To the Methodist way of thinking, Asclepiades represented the medical application of the atomic theories of Democritus and Epicurus, introduced to Rome by Lucretius (98–55 BC) in his poem, *De Rerum Natura* (On the Nature of Things), a work which was much in vogue in Rome at this time.[11]

In the view of Methodists, all diseases were governed by the same principles; they were divided into three basic physical states, two of which were excessively dry and constricted or excessively fluid and atomic. In the third state both conditions co-existed, comprising the famous *status strictus*, *status laxus* and *status mixtus* of Methodism. Their therapeutic principle was founded in *contraria contrariis*, i.e. 'relax the constricted, constrict the relaxed; when both states were present together, measures could be used that would attack the major disturbance without unduly aggravating the minor'. The approach was essentially methodic.[12] The basic doctrine of Methodism was cure by opposites; its purpose was to enlarge narrow pores and to reduce larger ones.

Asclepiades' therapies consisted of massage, exercise and cold-water bathing. He recommended swinging on a suspended couch, accompanied by food, wine and music. His slogan, *cito, tuto, jocunde* – 'swiftly, safely, sweetly' – is reflected in his therapies. Heroic venesection, much loved by those who practised classical medicine, he totally rejected. Both Pliny and Suetonius discuss cold-water baths. Apparently, Augustus, suffering from a 'dangerous illness' in 23 BC, which, according to Suetonius, was caused by abscesses on the liver, had his life saved by cold-water bathing. It was administered by his physician, Antonius Musa, a former slave and freedman of Mark Antony, who was himself a follower of Asclepiades.[13] Antonius Musa subsequently became wealthy as a result of his fame from curing the Emperor. However, even before this event, the doctor had cured Augustus of a more serious illness; for this he had been honoured with a statue, bought by public subscription and set up beside a statue of Asclepius. (Suet. *Aug.* 59). News of the cold-water cure spread from Rome to Marseilles:

> Charmis, also from Massilia, condemned not only previous physicians but also hot baths, persuading people to bathe in cold water even during the winter frosts. His patients he plunged into tanks, and we used to see old men, consulars, stiff with cold in order to show off.
>
> Pliny, *Nat. Hist.* 29.5.6–9

Self-styled Asclepiades flourished for three centuries. Galen, however, mocked their lack of philosophical reasoning and their use of pre-packed therapies.[14]

As already mentioned, one of the most important followers of the Methodist philosophy was Themison, a pupil of Asclepiades and a physician.

He was an original thinker who separated himself from his master and who formed a new method, centred on the observation of certain everyday symptoms of disease. He wrote the first systemic treatise on chronic disease. His lead was taken up by Thessalus of Tralles (c.AD 60) by whom the innovation was vigorously developed and flamboyantly[15] promoted, 'with a sort of rabid frenzy' (Pliny, *Nat. Hist.* 29.5.6-9) during the reign of the Emperor Nero (AD 54-68).

SORANUS OF EPHESUS

Soranus (*fl. c.*AD 100) was probably one of the greatest physicians of his day. Twenty-one works on a variety of subjects are attributed to him; they include surgery, *materia medica*, hygiene, ophthalmology, medical history and anatomy. Above all these, however, Soranus was an eminent authority on gynaecology and a prominent follower of Methodist medicine. Born in Ephesus in Asia Minor around the second half of the first century AD, he studied medicine at Alexandria, still a great centre of scientific enquiry at that time. Afterwards, in common with many Greek physicians, Soranus practised medicine at Rome. He died at about the time that Galen was born. Of all the works attributed to him, the most famous is the *Gynaecia*, arranged in four books. The work is practical in its outlook and consistent in its avoidance of superstition. One of his aims was to describe the physiological differences of male and female in the light of Methodist theory in which all diseases are governed by the same principles.

THE FOUR BOOKS OF THE GYNAECIA

Soranus uses the same names and headings as other Greek physicians when discussing clinical symptoms and the location of lesions; he is also interested in the cause, the aetiology, of a disease.[16] However, the Methodist distinction between *status laxus*, *status strictus* and *status mixtus* is always present:

> Now according to Methodist doctrine, the status is indicated by the symptoms as they develop in the course of the disease. It is easy to understand that diseases marked by a flux (for example gonorrhea: *Gynaecia* III.45) would be classified as belonging to the *status laxus* where a styptic treatment is indicated; whereas hysterical suffocation with its accompanying convulsions would impress the physician as presenting the *status strictus*, requiring a relaxing therapy.
>
> Temkin, *Introduction*, p.xxxii

Soranus' first book opens with a discussion of the different ways to describe gynaecology. This is best achieved by divisions into parts and sections, such as 'Theory and Practice', which is part hygiene and part therapy. The subject is also divided into 'Things Normal' and 'Things Abnormal' and into 'Physiology, Pathology and Therapy'. Soranus describes the qualities required in a midwife and the 'things with which the midwife is faced'. All these different perspectives serve to demonstrate the wide scope of Soranus' professional gynaecological practice.

Soranus is also concerned to explain in detail, 'What Persons Are Fit to Become Midwives?' One of the requirements (I.4) is that she should be free from superstition. He states that his purpose is to help others, by preventing their wasting time and trouble in teaching unfit persons:

> A suitable person will be literate, with her wits about her, possessed of a good memory and loving her work, respectable and generally not unduly handicapped as regards her senses, sound of limb, robust, and, according to some people, endowed with long slim fingers and short nails at her fingertips. She must be ... able to comprehend the art through theory, too ... so that she may easily follow what is said and what is happening; she must have a good memory to retain the imparted instructions ... She must love her work in order to persevere ... people will have to trust their household and the secrets of their lives to her ... these skills can be acquired through zealous endeavour and practice ...
>
> *Gynaecia*, III.3

In 'Things Normal' Soranus describes the female genitalia and the organs of reproduction. He includes a discussion of hygiene, normal pregnancy and labour, as well as infant care and children's illnesses. 'Things Abnormal' concerns women's diseases and their treatments. Soranus puts forward the question: 'Whether women have conditions peculiarly their own'. Although the enquiry is also bound up with philosophy, its main concern is with the subjects of anatomy, pathology and treatment. Indeed, it is a necessary question for Soranus to argue (III.2-3) because from it follows the problem concerning whether women need their own particular therapies. In support of his concept of women's diseases, Soranus advances the following opinions:

> We call some physicians women's physicians because they treat the conditions of women. And the public is wont to call in midwives in cases of sickness when the women suffer something peculiar which they do not have in common with men. Furthermore, the female is by nature different from the male ... Now that which is different in its whole nature will also be subject to its own diseases ... the uterus

is a part peculiar to women and the functions of the uterus appear in them alone, as menstruation, conception, parturition…

Gynaecia, III.2.3

In The Hippocratic treatise, 'Diseases of Women', the womb was thought to resemble a jar, in which the foetus could grow like a plant; and, like a jar, the womb had a mouth.[17] King[18] discusses ideas within the *Hippocratic Corpus* in which men and women differ. One of the main features which distinguished women from men is the presence of a route, a *hodos*, extending from the mouth and nostrils to the vagina, with a mouth at either end. Although no explicit anatomical description is given of this tube, it is possible to infer its existence from several references in the treatise. In addition to this belief, despite knowledge of the diaphragm, the womb was regarded as a separate entity which could roam around the body at will. However, both Soranus and Galen disagreed with these ideas. In antiquity *hysteria* referred to the painful sensations or feelings of suffocation which were attributed to movements of the womb. The word 'hysteria' has a different meaning today. With reference to Soranus' *Gynaecia* (IV.26) 'On hysterical suffocation', is best translated as 'suffocation of the womb'. Moreover, according to King,[19] 'hysteria is applied generally to female complaints'. In true Methodist style, a discussion of treatments given by other physicians, including any mistakes and faults that he may have found with them, is followed by Soranus' own therapeutic method. First the methods used by others:

But the majority of the ancients and almost all followers of the other sects have made use of ill-smelling odours (such as burnt hair, extinguished lamp wicks, charred deer's horn, burnt wool, burnt flock and skins, *castoreum* (an aromatic secretion obtained from the beaver) with which they anoint the nose and ears, pitch, cedar resin, bitumen, squashed bed bugs, and all substances which are supposed to have an oppressive smell, in the opinion that the uterus flees from evil smells. Wherefore they have also fumigated with fragrant substances from below, and have approved of suppositories of spikenard [and] storax, so that the uterus, fleeing the first-mentioned odours, but pursuing the last-mentioned, might move from the upper to the lower parts. Besides, Hippocrates made some of his patients drink a decoction of cabbage, others, asses' milk; he, believing that the uterus is twisted like the intestines are, when in intestinal obstruction, inserted a small pipe and blew air into the vagina by means of a blacksmith's bellows, thus causing dilation … Mantias gives *castroreum* and bitumen in wine to drink … he orders playing on the flute and drumming. Xenophon proposes torchlight and prescribes the making of greater noises by whetting and beating metal plates … Asclepiades … shouts loudly, and blows vinegar through the nose …

Such therapies as those described above could have had no place in Soranus' Methodist practice, in which women sufferering from abnormalities of the womb, or *hysteria*, would have benefited from a more relaxing treatment. On the same theme he continues:

> We, however, censure all these men who start by hurting the inflamed parts and cause torpor by the effluvia of ill-smelling substances... For the uterus does not issue forth like a wild animal from the lair, delighted by fragrant odours and fleeing bad odours; rather it is drawn together because of the stricture caused by the inflammation. Also upsetting the stomach, which suffers from sympathetic inflammation, and with toxic and pungent potions makes trouble. Forcing air by means of the smith's bellows into the vagina – this inflation makes the uterus more tense...
>
> *Gynaecia*, III.29

Almost by accident Soranus emerges as the main authority on the achievements of his predecessors. Their works now lost, his *Gynaecia* represents the body of knowledge gathered together up until the time of the early second century AD, albeit scrutinised and enlarged by Soranus.[20] In particular he admired Herophilus, according to whom, the uterus is woven from the same stuff as other parts and is affected in the same ways as them. Consequently, the Methodist view is, that there is no condition in women that can be regarded as particularly their own, except for those involving the organs of reproduction. The Asclepiadeans, of the same opinion, go further, contending that the female is composed of the same atoms as the male and becomes ill from the same causes, and is made well by the same therapies. Any differences between male and female are merely in their individual reproductive roles, all otherwise, concerning structure and function, is the same.

Contraception was practised in antiquity.[21] Soranus discusses the Hippocratic treatise 'On the Nature of the Child' in which the physician advises a girl to 'leap with the heels to the buttocks' in order to facilitate expulsion of an unwanted foetus. On the other hand, the Hippocratic Oath forbids giving a woman a drug for the purpose of procuring an abortion. In Soranus' opinion it is much more advantageous not to conceive than to destroy the embryo. He suggests a variety of measures that may be used to prevent conception. These range from the practice of *coitus interruptus* to the use of *materia medica*. The latter included the use of vaginal suppositories made from fine wool saturated in the juice of a fresh pomegranate, the peel of pomegranate (probably pounded) mixed in with its juice was another option. Oak galls, moist alum and Cimolian earth were used in this way, too. A vaginal application of pounded pomegranate peel with an equal amount of gum and oil of roses was another useful prescription. This was to be followed by a drink of honey water.

Moreover to some people this seems advisable: once during the month to drink Cyrenaic balm (from the silphium plant) to the amount of a chick-pea in two cyaths of water for the purpose of inducing menstruation. Or... panax balm and Cyreniac balm and rue seed, of each two obols, [grind] and coat with wax and give to swallow; then follow with a drink of diluted wine [or] wallflower seed and myrtle... or of white pepper... rocket seed or cow parsnip; drink with oxymel.

Gynaecia, I.62-3

All these things, according to Soranus, not only prevent conception, they also destroy any existing embryo. He discusses the use of amulets by some people but he says these ultimately reveal themselves as falsehoods.

ACUTE OR CHRONIC?

Another substantial treatise of Soranus in which Methodist principles are apparent is 'On Acute and Chronic Disease' which has come down to us in the Latin of Caelius Aurelianus who was a Methodist physician probably of the fifth or sixth century AD. Until the two states of acute or chronic disease were separated and described by the Methodist physician, diseases were not differentiated in this way. However, such classification was a good example of the patient-centred approach to medicine which the Methodists claimed to pursue, for it would have been of great service to diagnosis and treatment. As before, first the name and etymology of the disease was given, after which its chief characteristics and symptoms were listed. This was followed by prognosis and differentiation from other diseases.

Soranus defined acute diseases as those which terminate quickly and completely, with a good chance of spontaneous cure. Chronic diseases, by contrast, linger on and on. They are characterised either by periods of attack or intervals of remission, or repeated changes of visiting symptoms, according to the basic state that is involved, such as the predisposing factors, or the so-called manifest causes. Methodists, as already described, are not concerned with hidden causes. Chronic diseases require palliative care and the intervention of the physician, whose skills are greatly tested. Finally, in this treatise, the treatment is discussed, with again the naming of physicians and any former mistakes concerning each disease.

Some fifty diseases are discussed in detail. An example of one of these is apoplexy.[22] The name is derived from the Greek *pleso*, meaning 'strike'. It is always acute, never chronic. Soranus' description is clear, unemotional and immensely practical. The manifest sign is a sudden collapse. Soranus gives the predisposing factors.[23] These are: 'prolonged exposure to heat or violent cold, recurring indigestion aggravated by bathing; venery, especially in the case of old men; injury to the membrane of the brain and, in the case of children, violent jumping'. Some people receive warning signs, others do not. The disease may become worse, with a fatal conclusion, or it may be less severe, in which case recovery is possible, the cold numbness of the body giving way to warmth. The patient who recovers may suffer impairment of reason or speech. Soranus classifies apoplexy as a disease involving *status strictus*. He concludes the chapter with a description of the treatment.

The contribution of Methodism to medicine was in the stimulus it gave to accurate clinical observation.[24] However, because Methodism separated theory from practice, it was unable to progress when confronted with scientific medicine, which would have given the patient improved treatment.

MEDICAL PROVISION FOR THE MILITARY

During the Republic, the care of wounded and sick soldiers was organised on an *ad hoc* basis, but under Augustus and his successors other arrangements were necessary. The expansionist policies of the early Empire required soldiers to stay fit and healthy; they were also expected to fight in distant and hostile territories. In such circumstances, local householders could not be relied upon to give either medical care, or safe hospitality. As already described (chapter 4) a degree of self-sufficiency was eventually provided in the form of sick-bays or hospitals for soldiers who, due to the distances involved, could no longer return to their homes to be nursed back to health, as in former times. From this it follows that the establishment of a professional standing army and safe surroundings, *valetudinaria*, where the sick and wounded could be cared for, required the provision of medical services. The evolution of a military medical facility was a natural result following on from this need. Precise details of its organisation, however, are imperfectly understood, although a range of different posts is attested epigraphically. Vegetius (*Epitome* 2.10) states that the *praefectus castrorum* was responsible for the sick and for the *medici* 'by whom they were looked after and also all expenses involved'. Hospital administration was probably undertaken by the *optio valetudinarii*, who was also under the supervision of the *praefectus castrorum*. The most frequently attested title is *medicus*. Medical assistants were *milites medici* and *capsarii*. The doctors, *medici*, were composed from a variety of men of differing skills and experience and would probably have differed in rank and status.

The *medicus* was the medical officer under whom the dressers, *capsarii* (named after the *capsa*, the round bandage-box in which dressings were carried) worked. He would often have had a long career.[25] Davies cites Caius Papirius Aelianus who died at Lambaesis in Africa at the age of eighty-five years (*CIL* VIII, 18314 = *ILS* 2432) but still in service. The Roman Navy also had a medical provision, although its organisation, too, is unclear. It is, however, known from inscriptions that the Roman Navy was involved in building operations at Benwell, *RIB* 1340, and Hadrian's Wall between Birdoswald and Castlesteads, *RIB* 1944 and 1945. Axius, a *medicus ocularius* for the British Fleet (*Classis Britannica*, based at Dover) devised an eye-salve which according to Galen, writing in the second century AD, was quite effective and was likely to have been used widely. The ingredients were as follows: copper and zinc hydroxide, zinc carbonate, opium and mercuric sulphide; it was intended to be used on 'ulcered corners of the eye, bad inflammation of the eye, intense irritation and chronic condition of the eye'.[26]

The term *medicus ordinarius* is known on inscriptions throughout the Empire.[27] In each case, whether with legionary units or auxiliary, the holder of the post appears to have held Roman citizenship. Anicius Ingenuus, *medicus ordinarius* of the *Cohors 1 Tungrorum*, at Housesteads, on Hadrian's Wall (*CIL* VII, 690: = *RIB* 1618), who died at an early age of twenty-five years, would have been qualified according to the standards of the day. His tombstone, found in 1813, is now in Newcastle Museum (*88*). The carving on the buff limestone is quite elaborate and would have been relatively expensive. Ingenuus may

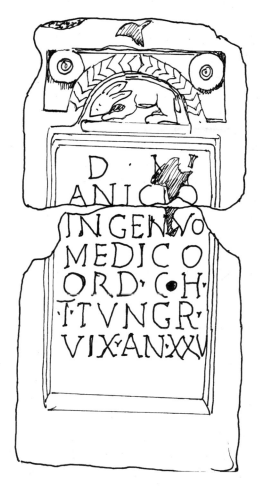

88 The tombstone of Anicius Ingenuus

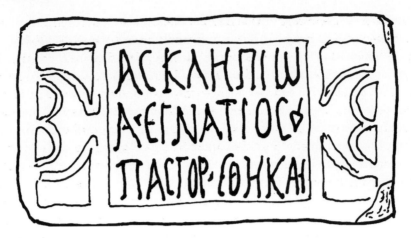

89 Dedication slab of Aulus Egnatius Pastor

have been a well-educated and skilled doctor who could have afforded to leave funds enough to pay for his monument, or else it was afforded by his family. An important point concerning this tombstone is the implication that the Roman health authorities treated all ranks equally where health was concerned. Both legionary and auxiliary garrisons alike would have been provided with hospitals and medical staff. Senior doctors were probably found above the rank of *medicus ordinarius*. They may have included those styled *medicus castrensis* or *medicus castrorum* (*CIL* XIII, 1883; VI, 31172).[28] At the fort at Vindolanda, the strength report shows that the medical staff there was caring for twenty to thirty soldiers classed as sick and wounded as well as those with infectious eye disease.

In Roman Britain, as elsewhere, religion and medical practice were not mutually exclusive and some doctors are known only from inscriptions which speak of their devotions to deities of healing. Altogether ten dedications to Aesculapius are known in Britain, some but not all, being on behalf of *medici*. A Greek inscription to Aesculapius from Maryport (*RIB* 808) was set up by Aulus Egnatius Pastor (*89*). He may have been a doctor.[29] Boon suggests that the dedicator could have been a freedman of the governor Egnatius Lucilianus. Doctors and their families enjoyed considerable mobility and might easily have been at the frontiers of Empire, as here.

M. Aurelius [Abr]ocomas, the doctor of the Cavalry Regiment of Vettonians at Binchester (*Vinovia*) in County Durham, erected a dedication slab depicting Aesculapius and Salus for the Cavalry Regiment, *Ala Vettonum Civium Romanorum* (*RIB* 1028). This probably dates to the third century. [Abr]ocomas seems to have been a Greek, for his name has a Greek termination (*90*). However, the point is that, without this inscriptional evidence, he would have remained unknown. Greek inscriptions are rare in Britain and at Chester a dedication by the doctor Hermogenes (*RIB* 461), erected to 'the mighty saviour gods', is a further reminder of the Greek origins of Roman medicine. It is interesting that Hadrian's doctor was also called Hermogenes.[30] This, however, is a name that was commonly used by doctors (*91*).

In 1968 another inscribed stone, that of a physician, Antiochus (*92*), was found a mere 70ft away from the above. This altar is the subject of an article[31] in which it is proposed that the conjunction of the two altars suggests that the doctors were attached to a fortress there. The close proximity of the find-spots may indicate that the residential area for army medical staff was situated in the *praetorium*. On the other hand, Webster[32] suggests that both stones were found in the area west of Northgate Street where there is evidence for what might have been a large *valetudinarium*. The presence of a *valetudinarium* at Chester has long been suspected, although none has so far been firmly identified. Like Hermogenes, Antiochus may well have been the personal physician of the Legionary Legate. However, the two altars of Hermogenes and Antiochus, inscribed in Greek, do not record the *tria nomina* indicative of Roman citizens, in either case. Therefore, it is possible that both men served at different times as the private physicians of the Legionary Legate. Finally, no firm evidence has been found to show that the Roman Army had commissioned surgeons or physicians. Neither is it certain[33] that *medicus ordinarius* implies a commissioned rank. Moreover, it is apparent from a treatment scene on Trajan's column where medical workers are seen bandaging wounds and wearing normal military dress, that ordinary soldiers were employed as medical personnel (*93*).

GALEN

The problem with Galen is that his voluminous output of philosophical and medical writings (more than 350 of his works are known)[34] makes it difficult

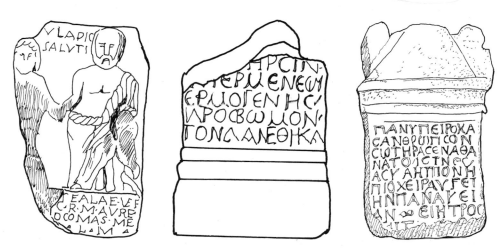

90 Left Dedication slab of Marcus Aurelius [...]ocomas, doctor; *91 Middle* Hermogenes' dedication on the lower part of an altar; *92 Right* The altar of Antiochus

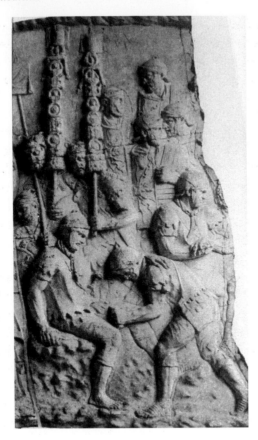

93 A field dressing station
portrayed on Trajan's
column

to decide where to begin a general discussion of his work. The first requirement, of course, is for biographical detail, but even here Galen is ambiguous,
for he was a clever self-publicist. He was well aware of what the background
of an up-and-coming young *medicus* should look like and he presented himself
accordingly.[35] Galen was born in AD 129, at Pergamum (now Bergama,
Turkey), where Roman rule had been established in the mid-second century
BC and an important temple of Asclepius had been built. He died AD 216?
in Rome (see Nutton, 2004). Coming from the Greek east, he wrote in
Greek and regarded himself as a Greek. It is possible that he did not learn
to speak Latin. In order to obtain the best medical education he travelled
extensively. Thereafter, most of his working life was spent in Rome. He left
Rome suddenly in 166, 'like a runaway slave', blaming his departure on the
animosity of his rivals. However, it is more probable that he wished to avoid
the plague which was raging at the time.

As the son of the wealthy architect and landowner, Nicon, Galen was
given the best of educations. He informs us that he studied philosophy until
his father experienced prophetic dreams concerning a future for his son in
medicine. Galen was fortunate in his relatives, for they tutored him in a liberal

education and by the age of fourteen he had been instructed by his father and grandfather in arithmetic, logic, geometry and grammar. By contrast, of his mother he writes, 'my mother... bit her serving maids and constantly shouted at my father'. Flemming[36] suggests that this fits in with classical patterns of self-presentation, where maleness is self-mastery and femaleness equals a lack of that quality. Moral guidance was taught to Galen by his father, both by his providing a 'shining example' and through direct advice. He informs us that his father advocated, 'with good effect', the virtues of the philosophers. These included justice, manliness, *sophrosyne* and intelligence, together with, the 'elevation of truth over glory' and control of the passions. However, as a result of the vivid dreams of Nicon, involving demands from Aesculapius, Galen became diverted from preparations for the philosophical life and was henceforward steered towards medicine.

Galen began his medical studies at the age of sixteen at Pergamum. He left Pergamum after his father's death in 148/9. He then travelled to Smyrna, Corinth and Alexandria, the most important centre for medical education. He returned to Pergamum in 157 and was appointed physician to the gladiators by the high priest. Galen records that the death-rate among gladiators became reduced as a result of his work and a complete cessation of fatalities was effected as a result of his continued stay.[37] Whilst in this post, Galen would have become experienced in the care of wounds, he could have observed internal organs in action and would have learnt much about diet, exercise and rehabilitation. By the time he travelled to Rome in 162, he was well known as a physician.

In the capital, Galen's high reputation increased. He claimed to dissect animals every day, practising in private in order to give good public performances. Galen diagnosed a case of love-sickness by observing the effect on the female patient when a certain dancer's name was mentioned. He cured the wife of Flavius Boethus of her flux after the 'best doctors in Rome' had failed to do so. Her husband was of consular rank and a friend of the Emperor; he thereafter became the friend and sponsor of Galen. His old philosophy tutor, Eudemus, suffered from a fever in the winter of AD 162-3, which other doctors had been unable to cure, and Galen was successful here, too.[38] He was now established as a fashionable healer and was employed in imperial service.

Galen's model of the body was based on the four humours: hot, cold, wet and dry. These are related to the fundamental substances of the universe (fire and water) and to the humours of the human body (blood, phlegm, yellow bile and black bile). For good health these needed to be in perfect balance and this was achieved through the correct *regimen*. Much of his writing involved dietetics, but he also included exercise, baths, massage and climate. Like Celsus, he was a great admirer of Hippocrates, from whom his model of the body was derived, in combination with Plato and Aristotle.[39] Galen composed many commentaries on the Hippocratic treatises. Although by this time the medical profession was divided into several mutually antagonistic sects, his own medical art was broad-based. He declared allegiance to no individual group, preferring to take from each what seemed to him to be right. After his death his influence caused the various sects to die out. However, ultimately Galen's dogmatism held up the course of scientific research for many centuries.[40]

THE PLAGUE OF JUSTINIAN

In the fourth century, the Roman Empire became divided, with capitals in Rome and Constantinople. The Eastern part endured until 1453 but the Western Empire was completely overrun in the fifth century. Under Justinian (527-65) the Greek portion was poised to bring its Latin counterpart back into the fold. Justinian's achievements in administrative reforms, his codification of Roman law, and the construction of the Church of Santa Sophia were well matched by his military achievements. However, his ambition to re-establish the unity of the Roman Empire was vanquished by disease, when the so-called 'Plague of Justinian' struck in the spring of 542. Justinian himself fell ill. Although he recovered, his imperial ambitions did not. This was the first plague pandemic. It was bubonic. The mortality and disruption caused by the plague prevented Justinian's restoration of the former extent of the Roman Empire.[41]

One of the symptoms of bubonic plague is the presence of buboes, swellings in the lymph nodes, which may be as large as an egg, or an orange. Once these swellings appeared, most sufferers would either pass into a deep coma, or they would become delirious, suffering from hallucinations and paranoia. As a result, great difficulty would be experienced when attempting to care for them, even when attempting to give food. Although the plague was first noticed in the Egyptian harbour town of Pelusium, the causative bacillus appears to have originated in central Africa and India, the probable home of the black rat which carried the plague bacillus, *Yersinia pestis*, in its blood. Once a person is infected with *Y. pestis*, the lymphatic system reacts to collect the infection and bubonic swellings result from this reaction. The plague may also assume a pneumonic phase, in which case infection is transmitted in the saliva, or in coughing. In these cases the infection bypasses the rats and fleas and moves directly between humans. The pathogen may also be blood-borne (septicaemic), in which case the lymphatic system becomes overwhelmed. The plague was described in detail by Procopius of Caesarea in his *History of the Wars*:

> During these times there was a pestilence, by which the whole human race came near to being annihilated... For this calamity it is quite impossible either to express in words or to conceive in thought

any explanation, except indeed to refer it to God. For it did not come in a part of the world nor upon certain men, nor did it confine itself to any season of the year, so that from such circumstances it might be possible to find subtle explanations of a cause, but it embraced the entire world, and blighted the lives of all men, though differing one from another in the most marked degree, respecting neither sex nor age. For much as men differ with regard to places in which they live, or in active pursuits, or in whatever else man differs from man, in the case of this disease alone the difference availed naught. And it attacked some in the summer season, others in the winter, and still others at the other times of the year. Now let each one express his own judgement concerning the matter, both sophist and astrologer, but as for me, I shall proceed to tell where the disease originated and the manner in which it destroyed men.

Procopius, II.xxi–ii.1–7

The disease may have spread northwards to Britain in 544, for in the late seventh century the Venerable Bede writes of a sudden plague which had first decimated the southern parts of Britain and later spread northwards, eventually reaching Ireland. It may also be possible to discern a reference to plague in the quotation from Gildas, given below. The Plague of Justinian is significant for, like the Plague of Athens almost a millennium before, it marked the end of a particular way of life. Now came the close of the Classical world and the beginning of the Dark Ages, as pestilences followed one after another during the next 200 years. All was not quite dark, however. Although Roman rule may have come to an end, two important texts, each having relevance to medicine, demonstrate the possibility that Roman government in Britain continued. As already implied, the text of Gildas, written *c.*AD 540 (probably in south-west Britain), perhaps unwittingly, carries intimations of plague. The value of the text in this context is that it demonstrates continuity of Roman cultural values in Britain. Gildas' *De Excidio Britonum*, 108.1–2:[42]

What further? I bring before you to confound you the example of Mathias [and the holy apostles]; he drew his lot not at his own will, but by the choice and judgement of Christ. Yet you are blind to this instance, and do not see how far removed you are from his merits: for you have rushed headlong and of your own volition into the greed and disposition of the traitor, Judas. It is clear, then, that anyone who calls you priest knowingly and from his heart, is no excellent Christian. I will tell you what I feel. My reproach might be gentler; but what is the point of merely stroking a wound or smearing it with ointment when it already festers with swelling and stink, and requires cautery and the public remedy of fire? – if indeed it can be cured at all when the sick man is not looking for a cure and shrinks away from this doctor.

The following inscription (*94*) almost contemporary with the text of Gildas, was recorded on a monument dedicated to a doctor and found in a churchyard in Llangian, Caenarvonshire, Gwynedd:[43]

MELI MEDICI

FILI MARTINI

IACIT

The translation reads, 'The stone of Melus, doctor, son of Martinus. He lies here'. The inscription suggests that even at this late date in the history of Roman Britain it may be possible to view the presence of a *magistratus* and a doctor in north Wales as demonstrating an ordered system of government, with Roman medicine continuing, at least in one part of Britain.[44]

CONCLUSION

The Hippocratics (*95*) formed the basis of preventative medicine through their theories concerning diet and exercise, or *regimen*. Moving on to Roman medicine, we find healing going on at different levels. There was a good understanding of herbal medicine and simple surgery, the latter leading to the development of attractive and functional surgical tools. At the same time, temple medicine informs us of the areas of concern that most occupied the minds of Romans. Furthermore, Roman improvements in water supply led to the provision of public baths and the proper disposal of sewage, giving improved standards of hygiene. All this was combined with an active interest to find out more about the way the human body worked.

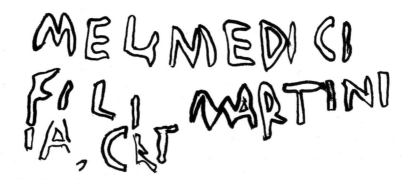

94 An inscription from Late Roman Britain

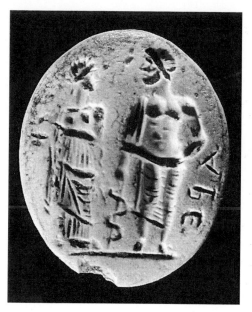 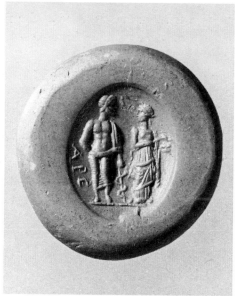

95 A cornelian intaglio found at Braintree, Essex, showing Asclepius and Hygea. The inscription is cut in retrograde to give the positive impression 'APE' – perhaps rendered 'Virtue' and alluding to the Hippocratic Oath. The gemstone would have been set in a ring and perhaps was owned by a doctor

The wonders of modern surgery are due to a more complete understanding of anatomical and physiological processes, the advent of chemotherapy and the possibility for finely tuned anaesthesia, none of which was available in antiquity. In modern times international programmes of vaccination and immunisation have helped to greatly reduce many of the killer diseases such as tuberculosis, poliomy-elitis, anthrax and diphtheria. In the late nineteenth century the cause of malaria was established, when it was found to be due to the transmission of parasites by mosquitoes. In the 1930s and 1940s that disease became largely eradicated from southern Europe.[45] Moreover, radiography and radiology have vastly improved aids to diagnosis and treatment. This is all positive and good, indeed, it is tempting to believe that medicine can do almost anything and that Pandora's box has been replaced by the treasure-chest of science.

However, implicit in all these improvements comes a health warning, for it has been argued elsewhere that progress itself is a disease-forming agent.[46] Deadly bacteria and viruses continue to mutate and to attack vulnerable people, particularly those with lowered immunity, as they enter crowded places where it is possible for pathogens to collect. This includes hospitals, artificially ventilated public-transport systems and places of entertainment. In addition to new pathogens, known as 'super-bugs', many of the old illnesses, such as tuberculosis, assumed to have been vanquished, are returning. Indeed, patients entering hospital today, in particular those who are already coping with the stresses of chronic disease, face the possibility of contracting any one of several potentially lethal infections, of types that could never have been encountered in antiquity.[47]

EPILOGUE

In this discussion of Roman medicine it has been shown that a degree of knowledge and practice was inherited from earlier heritages of Hellenistic writings and to this Rome added her own innovations. However, when in the fourth century AD, the Western empire collapsed, the impetus for medical progress passed to the east, the chief catalyst being the spread of Christianity. Conflicts arising between Christians of different sects, as they disputed over dogma and creed in Byzantium, caused the enforced exile of large numbers of Christian scholars (many of whom were physicians) to the easternmost provinces. This resulted in a resurgence of intellectual life in Edessa, a city well placed for people travelling on the Silk Routes to China. The position of the city, at the centre of the trade crossroads, favoured the growth of a group of cultured merchants. Many of these would have played an important role in the development and distribution of medicinal substances. Christian scholars spread to the East throughout Persia, as far as Samarkand and beyond. They established schools with libraries and hospitals with the provision of medical services. Ancient manuscripts, including the medical texts of Galen, Dioscorides and Celsus, were carried there and translated from Greek into Syriac, a language which combines elements of Aramaic and Greek. Hellenic learning in medicine, philosophy and the sciences took on a form not very distant from its origins, but with an increasingly non-Hellenic cast. The atmosphere was one in which scholarship could flourish. Eventually, by the time of the early medieval period, an industrious period of translating Greek and Latin texts into Arabic began and large teaching hospitals appeared in Islamic countries. However, all that belongs to another subject and another time and this account of Roman medicine ends here.

ABBREVIATIONS

AA	*Archaeologia Aeliana*
ANRW	*Aufstieg und Niedergang der Römischen Welt*
Ant.	*Antiquity*
Ant. J.	*Antiquaries Journal*
Arch. J.	*Archaeological Journal*
BAR	*British Archaeological Reports*
B.G.	*Caesar*, De Bello Gallico
BHM	*Bulletin of the History of Medicine*
Brit.	*Britannia*
CIL	*Corpus Inscriptionum Latinum*
CSIR	*Corpus Signorum Imperii Romani*
ET	*Edelstein Testimonies*
GMM	*Greenwich Medical Media, London*
IJO	*International Journal of Osteoarchaeology*
JCAS	*Journal of the Chester Archaeological Society*
JRA	*Journal of Roman Archaeology*
JAS	*Journal of Archaeological Sciences*
JBAA	*Journal of the British Archaeological Association*
JRSM	*Journal of the Royal Society of Medicine*
JRS	*Journal of Roman Studies*
LCL	*Loeb Classical Library*
Med. Hist.	*Medical History*
Nat. Hist.	*Pliny the Elder*, Naturalis Historia
P. Soc. Ant. Scot.	*Proceedings of the Society of Antiquaries of Scotland*
RCHMC	*The Royal Commission on Historical Monuments*
RIB	*R.G. Collingwood and R.P. Wright,* The Roman Inscriptions of Britain
SAMJ	*South African Medical Journal*
TBGAS	*Transactions of the Chester Archaeological Society*
WAM	*Wiltshire Archaeological Magazine*

Acknowledgements for illustrations, drawings and maps

Courtesy of the National Museums and Galleries on Merseyside, Liverpool, cover plate and *49*

Robin Gray, *3* and *19*

Roz Park, *16, 18* and *colour plate 9*

Courtesy of the Trustees of the British Museum, London, *32, 47, 50, 51, 61, 69, 81a*

Courtesy of Mark Hassall, *95*

Courtesy of the Ashmolean Museum, Oxford, *26, 72a*

Simon Cruse, courtesy of Ralph Jackson, *41, 43, 64, 71b* and *c; colour plates 19, 26, 29, 31, 33, 34*

Courtesy of Bob Arnott, *colour plate 1*

From the estate of the late T.F.C. Blagg, *54*

The Journal of the British Archaeological Association, 57 and *58*

Jennie Cruse, *colour plate 11*

Courtesy of York Archaeological Trust, *colour plate 22*

Marjorie Cruse, *6* (after Ugolini in Bergmann, Johannes, 1998); *23, 24* and *29* redrawn from Mann 1999 (but *23* ultimately derived from Bentley and Triman, 1830); *21* and *29* (derived from *Medicinal Planzar*, Koehler, pub. Mumford); *28* (derivation unknown). Clive Coward at the Wellcome picture library kindly tracked down all the early references; Drawing *30* is after an illustration in the 'Vienna Dioscorides'

Philip Briant, *colour plates 14, 20a*

David Kelly, *35, 36, 37*

Barry Hobson, *34*

Gerald Hart, *66*, courtesy of Viscount Bledisloe, Lydney Park, Glos.

Jennifer Wakely, *82, 83, 84, 85a* and *b, 86*

Bruno Loreti, *56*

Courtesy of Gaspare Baggieri, *53, 72b*

Courtesy of Mathieu Giles, Conservateur du Musée Départmental d'art ancien,

Epinal, France, *colour plate 21*

Denise Allen, Andante Travels, *colour plate 24*

Courtesy of Philip Crummy, Colchester Archaeological Trust, *colour plates 30a and b*

Courtesy of TAP, Greek Ministry of Culture, *colour plates 7, 8*

The Wellcome Institute Picture Library, *2, 13, 17, 80*

Courtesy of Roger Tomlin, *22, 48*

Norfolk Museums and Archaeology Service, *78*

Society of Antiquities of London, *65*

Martin Henig, *33, 40, 59, colour plate 28*

Insititue of Archaeology, Oxford, *21, colour plates 10, 32*

Museum of Archaeology and Anthropology, Cambridge, *42*

Phillipa Content, *colour plates 4, 5, 6*

David Gilbert *48a*

Lastly many thanks are extended to John Steane for his fine drawings at numbers:, *20, 31a and b, 46, 52, 60, 62, 63, 67, 68, 70, 71, 73, 74, 75, 77, 79, 87, 88, 89, 90*

Remaining photographs and figures are the work of the author.

NOTES

INTRODUCTION

1   Hippocrates, 1st Aphorism: 'Life is short, the art of medicine is long; opportunity fleeting, experiment dangerous, judgement difficult. It is not enough for the physician to do what is necessary but the patient and the attendants must do their part too; circumstances must also be favourable.'
2   Porter, 1997, p.71
3   King, 2002, p.5
4   Porter, 1997, p.64
5   Miller, J.I., *Spice Trade*, chapters 9 and 13
6   King, 1998, p.7

I. GREEK CULT AND MEDICINE

1   Hesiod, *Works and Days*, ln.60–110 and 101-4, trans., M.L. West
2   Aeschylus, *Prometheus Bound*, ln.478-83, trans., Philip Vellacott
3   Majno, 1975, p.146; Hood, 1978, 108/9 and 253 n.16
4   *ibid.*, pp.145-6
5   Beaumann, 1983, p.19
6   Lucian, *Satirical Sketches*, p.26, trans. Paul Turner; in which the rival claims of literary culture are contrasted with the *techne* of sculpture, to the disadvantage of the latter
7   Majno, 1975, p.143
8   King, 1998, p.72
9   Majno, 1975, p.143
10 *ibid.*, p.152
11 Hart, 2000, has many references to serpents, particularly pp.46-7
12 Kerényi, 1960, pp.28-30 and 59 (kŭvás = of a dog)
13 Tomlinson, R.A., 1983, pp.7-94
14 Levi, Peter, *Pausanias: Guide to Greece*, Vol.1. p.195, Nos.160;198
15 *ibid.*, Vol.1. p.192
16 *ibid.*, Vol.2. p.194
17 See also chapter 5, note 65
18 King, 1998, p.106
19 Levi, Peter, *Pausanias: Guide to Greece*, Vol.1. p.193; ET, No.532
20 *ibid.*, Vol.1. p.193; ET, No.533
21 *ibid.*, Vol.1. p.492; ET, No.536
22 Plato, *Phaedo*, 118a, Penguin (ed.), p.183

23 Levi, Peter, *Pausanias: Guide to Greece*, Vol.1. pp.97-9
24 Petracos, Basil, *The Amphiareion of Oropos*, p.49
25 Melas, Evi, *Temples and Sanctuaries of Ancient Greece*, pp.29-37

2. GREEK SCIENCE AND MEDICINE
1 Murray, 1993, pp.21-28 and 249-51
2 Aristophanes parodied the Sophists in his play, *The Clouds*
3 Nutton, 1995
4 Temkin, 1953
5 *World of Athens*, 1984 (Open University Course Book), p.81
6 Thucydides, trans. Rex Warner
7 King, 2001, p.23
8 Poole, J.F.C. & Holladay, A.J., 1979
9 Lloyd, Geoffrey E.R., (ed.), 1978, p.249, trans. Chadwick & Mann
10 *ibid.*, p.71
11 *ibid.*, p.276
12 Nunn, 1996, p.122
13 Mann, 1992, p.121
14 *ibid.*, pp.142-3
15 Nunn, 1996, pp.29-30
16 *ibid.*, pp.176-7

3. MATERIA MEDICA, OR THE MATERIALS OF MEDICINE
1 Entralgo, p.116
2 Gordon, Richard, 1992, p.366; King, 1986
3 Gordon, Richard, 1992, p.373
4 *RIB* 11.3.2423.1; Henig *Corpus*, No.369
5 Tomlin, *Britannia* Vol. XXVII, 1996, pp.443-6
6 Information from Martin Henig
7 Gibbins, D., 1997.
8 Nijus, K., 1995, p.50
9 Sherratt, Andrew, 1996
10 Penn, R.G., 1994, pp.78-90
11 Murray, O., 1993, pp.122-3
12 King, 1988, pp.50-53
13 Scarborough, 1995
14 Scarborough, 1995, p.5; Riddle, J., 1985, pp.94-131
15 Scarborough, 1995, p.8
16 Jackson, 1992b, pp.44-5
17 Youti, Louise C., Michigan Medical Codex. Introduction by Ann Ellis Hanson, 1996, and pp.33-46, 47, 55, 73
18 Singer, Charles, 1927, pp.34-5
19 Flemming, Rebecca, 2000, p.43
20 Jashemski, W.F., 1999, pp.1-22
21 Ciaraldi, Marina, 2000
22 Riddle, 1985, pp.53, 62, 146
23 Ciaraldi, Marina, 2000, p.5
24 Majno, 1975, pp.413-7
25 Petronius, *The Satyricon*, trans., J.P. Sullivan
26 Godwin, 1974, p.480
27 *Current Archaeology*, No.150
28 *RIB* 2494.94
29 *JRS* 53, 1963, No.51, Davies, 1970b, 94, fig.10

4. ROMAN HEALTH AND HYGIENE: THE BUILDINGS

1 Strabo, *The Geography* (5.3.8.), cited in Potter, 1987, p.140
2 Evans, Harry B., 1994, *Water Distribution in Ancient Rome: the evidence of Frontinus*, The University of Michigan Press, Ann Arbour, paperback edition, 1997: contains full bibliography and notes; Smith, Norman, 1978, 'Roman Hydraulic Technology' in *Scientific American*, 1978, No.238, pp.154-161; Scobie, Alex, 1986, *Slums, Sanitation and Mortality in the Roman World*, *KLIO*, 68, 2, pp.399-433
3 Evans, p.137
4 *ibid.*, p.135
5 Vitruvius, *The Ten books on Architecture*, trans. M.H., Morgan, 1914, Dover Publications
6 Cited in Jackson, 1988, p.45
7 Inscription found in H. Bloch, 1944; Evans, pp.130-1; Jackson, 1988, pp.43
8 *ibid.*, pp.140-1
9 Scobie, 1986, p.402, fn.25
10 *ibid.*, p.416 but no ref. for inscription
11 *ibid.*, p.417 among others, Juv. *Sat.*1. p.131
12 Cited in Scobie, 1986, p.420, fn.161, *Laudatio muscae* p.4
13 Jackson 1988, pp.53, fn.80; Celsus, *De Med.* XI.8, pp.30-3
14 *Current Archaeology*, 1997, No.154, pp.363-369, source Bill Putnam, *The Dorchester Roman Aquaduct*
15 Boon, 1974, pp.86 and 103
16 Celsus VI.6.10; Galen, XII, 786K; Celsus IV.26.3-4; refs. cited in Jackson, 1988, p.47
17 Scobie, p.413
18 Aelian 13.6
19 Attested by Varro, 1.13.4.; Columella 1.6.24.; 10. 84f; 11.3.12, ref. in Scobie, p.414
20 Millet & Graham, 1986, pp.130-1, No.491, fig.91
21 Jansen, Gemma, 1997, pp.121-33
22 Martial, *Epigrams* XI.lxxvii.1-3, 'For hours, for a whole day, he'll sit/ On every public lavatory seat./ It's not because he needs a shit:/ He wants to be asked out to eat'
23 Knights, Dickson, Dickson & Breeze, 1983, *Journal of Archaeological Science*, 10, pp.139-52, 'Evidence concerning the Roman Military Diet at Bearsden, Scotland, in the second century AD'
24 Wacher, 1994, p.138
25 Addyman, 1989, p.246-8
26 In Boon 1983, fn.80, 'At York, spicules of marine sponges used instead of toilet paper were found in the sewer – the first instance of the well-known literary reference is archaeologically borne out
27 Delaney, 1999, p.67-74
28 Dunbabin, p.8, see also pp.30 and 33-9
29 Koenen, C., 1904, 'Beschreibung von Novaesium', *Bonner Jahrbücher* 111/112: pp.97-242
30 Baker, Patricia A., 2002, *The Roman Military Valetudinaria: fact or fiction?* pp 1-28; 'Medical care for the Roman Army on the Rhine, Danube and British Frontiers in the first, second and early third centuries AD', PhD Thesis, Chapter 6, Questioning the identification of the *valetudinaria*, pp.180-236
31 *ibid.*
32 Davies, 1989, p.218
33 Liversidge, 1968; Webster, 1960; Nutton, 1969; Majno, 1975; Johnson, 1983; Jackson, 1988; Davies, 1989
34 Davies, 1989, notes 80-101, pp.295
35 Dyczek, P., 1995; Press, Ludwika, 1988, *Valetudinaria at Novae and other Roman Danubian Hospitals*
36 Baker, Patricia A., 'Pollution and Magic: Cultural Concepts and Variations in Attitudes towards Roman-style medical Tools', Taboo, unpublished lecture

37 Fitzpatrick, *Britannia*, 1991, pp.143-6
38 Pitts & St Joseph, 1985
39 Boon, 1987
40 Bosanquet, 1904; Wilson, 1972; Charlesworth, 1976; Crow, 1995
41 Bowman, Alan K., 1994, pp.13-42; Bowman & Thomas, 1991, pp.62-74; Bowman & Thomas, 1994, pp.98-100, 204, 291
42 Bowman & Thomas, 1994, Doc.156, p.100
43 *ibid.*, 1991, Doc.154, p.69
44 I am grateful to Professor Alan Bowman for giving me a copy of the list written on this tablet, together with analysis, prior to publication
45 Youtie, Louise C., 1996, pp.76-7
46 Tomlin, *Britannia* xxii, 1991, No.24, p.299, fn.35
47 Gask & Todd, 1953, pp.126-8
48 St Jerome, *Epistulae*, LXXVII, 4.45

5. ROMAN DISEASES AND HEALING I: CULT

1 Karlen, 1996, pp.37-9
2 Salares, 2002, p.50
3 Jackson, 1988, pp.10-11
4 Potter, T.W., *JBAA*, 1985, p.37
5 Girardon, 1993, p.32
6 Wheeler & Wheeler, 1933
7 Painter, K., *JSA*, L, 1971, Vol.LI, Part 11, pp.329-31, and plate LXVII
8 *RIB* 2246.9-10 and 18
9 Baggieri, 1998, p.790
10 Dalrymple, 1998, pp.189-9
11 Blagg, 1986; Ann Inscher 'Discovering Nemi session', at Brewhouse Yard Museum, Nottingham
12 When permission was given by the owner for excavation of the site, it was on condition that the artefacts would be shared, and that the owner should choose what he wanted for himself; these objects were sold to dealers etc. Therefore, those artefacts shipped back to Nottingham were not representative of the total types of finds
13 Refs from Blagg, 1986, 218: Catullus' poem 3; Ovid *Fasti* iii.266; Statius *Silvae* III, pp.55-60
14 Blagg, 1986, p.211
15 *Ibid.*, p.218
16 Statius, *Silvae* III, pp.55-60, ref. in Blagg, 1986, p.218
17 Potter, 1987, pp.179
18 Plut. Sull.6; *CIL*.i.569
19 Servius, in Virg. *Georg.* III; refs. in Blagg, 1986
20 Frazer, 1890, p.141
21 Blagg, 1986, p.21
22 All archaeological information regarding the site comes from the work of the late Dr. T.W. Potter, pub. *JBAA*, cxxxviii (1985), pp.23-47, and plates vi-xi
23 A small group of anatomical votives from Veii may be seen in the Pitt-Rivers Museum in Oxford. Information from Dr. Martin Henig
24 Dionysius of Halicarnassus, ref. in Salares 2002, p.4
25 Salares, pp.259-60, fn.63
26 Von Staden, 1991
27 Salares, 2002, p.41
28 Pedley, 1990, pp.40-41
29 *Ibid.*, pp.75, 88 and 125. Also Ammerman & Cipriani in *AJA*, vol.101, 1997, p.347
30 Anonymous *On Famous Men*, 22.1.1-3, trans. Lewis & Reinhold, vol.1, in Chisholm &

Fergusson, 1981

31   Suet., *Claud.* 25

32   Dr Martin Henig reminds me that this was a divine space in which it would have been natural for kind individuals to set up to heal; thus a connection with a hospital could have followed

33   The Royal Hospital of St Bartholomew, 1123-1973, eds Medvei & Thornton, p.20, pub., 1974

34   The British Medical Journal, Vol. 11 for 1895, under the title, *Donatia of* Medical Interest

35   Hart, 2000, pp.111-13; Penn 1994,37-9

36   Jackson, 1988 fn.10, p.195; Republican epidemics: Livy, *History of Rome*, XXXIX, 41; XL,19,6-8 and 36,13-37,7; XLI,21,5-10. Epidemic of AD 65: Suetonius, *Nero* 39.1. Epidemic of AD 189: Cass. Dio, LXXII.14.3-4

37   Karlen,1996, pp.70-71

38   Jackson, 1988, p.172

39   *Ibid.*, 1988, p.174

40   Barker, 1997, pp.215-6

41   *RIB* 281

42   Bagnall-Smith, 1996, p.181

43   Painter, K.S., 1971, 'A Roman gold ex-voto from Wroxeter, Shropshire' *Ant.J.*L1, pp.329-31

44   Barker, 1997, pp.212-6

45   Wedlake, 1982; Henig, 1984, pp.131, 162

46   E.III No.1741, Liversidge, 1968, pp.335 and fn.3

47   Green, M.J., 1983, pp.51-3

48   Barnes, 1914, p.81

49   *RJ*, 1988, p.163

50   Jackson, *ibid.*

51   Examples include *RIB* Nos 1078, 1079, 1080 and 1081 from Lanchester

52   *RIB* 1052

53   *RIB* 218

54   *RIB* 319

55   *RIB* 126

56   Green, M.J., 1983, pp.16, 47

57   Wheeler & Wheeler, 1932, p.89, and pl.xxvi, No.121. The site and the museum are open to the public Sundays, Wednesdays, and Bank Holiday Mondays, from late March until early June

58   Personal communication from Martin Henig

59   Boon, 1989

60   *RIB* 305, *RIB* 306 and *RIB* 307

61   *RIB*, 616 and 617

62   Henig, 1984, 55, No.46

63   Hart, 2000, p.159

64   Edelstein's Testimonies 423.20 and 26 for a curative dog's lick: 'Lyson of Hermione, a blind boy. While wide-awake he had his eyes cured by one of the dogs in the Temple and went away healed'. 'A dog cured a boy from Aegina. He had a growth on the neck. When he had come to the god, one of the sacred dogs healed him – while he was awake – with its tongue and made him well'

65   Hart, 2000, p.98

66   Wheeler & Wheeler, 1932, p.89, and pl.xxvi, No.121

67   Henig, 1984, p.136

68   *Coll. rerum mem.* (ed.) Mommsen (1985) p.102

69   Cunliffe & Davenport, 1985, 130 No.9a

70   Henig, 1984, 43, 135, and 153

71   *CSIR*, Vol.1, Fasc.2, No.3, pl.ii

72   Bartlett, 991; Frere 1990. Information kindly supplied by Bagnall-Smith

73   Huskinson, *CSIR*, Vol.1, No.11, pl.iv, p.6. and Green, M.J., 1976, p.220

74   Henig in Woodward & Leach, 107, 1 and 108, pl.94, 1

75 Tomlin, Roger
76 Frankfurter, 1998, Taks, 1994
77 Frankfurter, David, 1998, p.163; Montserrat, 1998
78 Takács, Sarolta, 1994
79 Kenneth Painter kindly sent me a print-out of his lecture presented at Rewley House to the Oxford Archaeological and Historical Society, Feb. 2001
80 Information from the website for Fieldwork in Israel 20/09/01, created and maintained by Richard Baylis, Museum of Antiquities, University of Newcastle upon Tyne
81 Dr. Gerald Hart kindly provided the information concerning this discovery

6. ROMAN DISEASES AND HEALING II: 'MEDICAMENTS, CAUTERIES AND OPERATIONS'

1   Künzl, Ernst, 1991, in *The Celts: the origins of Europe*, p.372
2   Jackson, 2002, p.88
3   Galen, II.68.2, Khun. ref. cited in Jackson, 1988, p.114
4   Jackson, 2002b
5   Jackson, 2002a, p.89
6   Jackson, 1993, p.80: Personal communication from Ralph Jackson
7   Hippocrates, *De Decenti Habitu* 8.10-13 (9.236-238L) ref. cited in Jackson, 2002, p.91
8   Jackson, 1994, p.168
9   Jackson, 1994; Majno 1975, pp.359 and 361, ill. 9.14 and 9.15
10 Jackson, 1988, p.197
11 Boon, 1974, p.137
12 Jackson, 2002a, p.90
13 Until recently, medical or surgical instruments had attracted interest amongst only a small number of scholars. The renewal of interest in them and in the archaeology of medicine in general, which has occurred over the past twenty years, is a result of more evidence being available from an increased number of finds and of the development of new ways of looking and thinking about the subject. Formerly it seems to have been generally assumed that the paucity of evidence meant that such a study would not be worthwhile. A few useful publications do exist, however. One of the earliest is by a practising surgeon, J.S. Milne, in 1907, which remains useful. Moreover, recent publications are to hand, such as the articles and smaller catalogues, mostly written and illustrated by Ralph Jackson at the British Museum, who is the leading authority in the field in Britain. Other scholars have also contributed important works to the subject of Roman medical and surgical instruments. Notable works include Künzl (1983; 1996); Krug (1985); Bliquez (1994) and Jackson (1986; 1990; 1994a)
14 Jackson, 1986, *Brit.* 17, pp.119-67
15 Jackson, 2002a, p.90
16 Jackson, 1997d
17 Crummy, 1997; Jackson, 1997b and 1997c
18 Jackson 2002a, p.91 (refs in Jackson: Maiuri, 1939, pp.218-21; Künzl, 1983, pp.12-15; Bliquez, 1994, pp.87-8, 207-8)
19 Jackson 2002a, p.91
20 Jackson, 1990, p.10
21 Jackson, 2002, p.89
22 Jackson, 1990, p.10
23 Jackson, 1994, p.332, and 1997d, p.16
24 Bliquez, L.J., 1992, pp.35-50
25 E. Künzl, 1982, 114-5, fig. 4 and Ralph Jackson, 1994b, 325-32
26 Bliquez, *PACT*, 34, 1992, pp.35-50
27 Bliquez, pp.43-4
28 Henig, 1984, pp.20 and 187
29 Boon, in Zienkiewicz, *Caerleon* 11, 159
30 Bliquez, 1992, p.44

31   Rossitsa Nenova-Merdjanova, 1999, *JRA* pp.130-4

32   Bliquez, p.43

33   *ibid.*, p.44

34   Bellamy & Pfister, 1992, p.7: Sherratt, 1996b

35   Jackson, 1995, p.198

36   For trephination see: Brothwell, D., Powers, R., & Denston, B. *WAM.* 70/71, 1978, pp.43-60; Brothwell, D. *JAS*, 1, 1974, pp.209-11; Wells, C. *Antiquity*, 1974, 48, pp.298-300; Parker, S. & Manchester, K.A. *OSSA*, 1986, 12, pp.141-158; McKinley, J.I. *IJO*, Vol.2, pp.333-5, 1992 and *IJO*, pp.341-9

37   Jackson, 1992a, p.168

38   *ibid.*, p.168

39   *ibid.*, p.170

40   *ibid.*, p.75

41   Jackson & Leahy, 1990

42   Boon, 1874, p.137

43   Jackson, 1997c

44   Crummy, 1996a, pp.1-9

45   Stead, 1967, pl.1, pp.16-19

46   Henig, 1984, p.39

47   N.P. Wickenden in *Britannia*, 17, 1986, pp.348-51

48   Crummy, *Current Archaeology*, 1997

49   Stead, 1967, pp.23-5, pl.V a, b, c, and fig.13

50   Crummy, 1977, 18; 2002, p.47-57

51   Megaw & Megaw, 1989, pp.160-6

52   Jackson, 1997c

53   Boon 1974, p.137

54   Boon 1974, 124, fig.9

55   Gilson, 1981, p.6

56   Gilson, 1982 and 1988

57   Jackson, 1986, pp.154-5

58   Lindsay Allason-Jones 1979, pp.239-41

59   Wells, *Ant*.41, pl.xvii, b.1967, pp.139-41

60   Wheeler, R.E.M., No.3, 1930, reprinted 1946, pp.79-83, pls.XXXVII and XXXVIII

61   Personal communication from Jackson (in my MA dissertation)

62   Jackson, 1996a, pp.2243-2250; 2002, p.92

63   Boon (1983/4)

64   Jackson, 1988, p.82

65   ref. in Boon, 1983

66   Künzl, 1985; Jackson, 1996b

67   Nutton, 1972

68   Jackson, 1996b (see map, after Jackson 1996b. p.178, fig.21.1)

69   Jackson, 1996

70   Jackson, 1996b, 180

71   Boon, 1983, p.1-2

72   Jackson, 1992b

73   Potter, 1978 in Jackson 1996b

74   Jackson, 1997b, p.180

75   Jackson, 1996b

76   Jackson, 1997b

7. MEETING THE ROMAN PATIENT

1   The coin-image of Marcus Aurelius was provided courtesy of the British Museum. For references to Marcus Aurelius as a patient see Jackson 1988, pp. 61, 64, 70, 146, 162, 170, 173, 174

2 Stirland, A. & Waldron,T., 1990, pp.221-30
3 Wells, Calvin, 1973
4 Wenham, L., 1968; Harman, M., Molleson, T.I., Price, J.L., 1981; Waldron, T., 1995; Wakely, J., 1996
5 McWhirr, Viner & Wells, 1982, pp.161-72
6 Johnston, Francis E., 1963 also Darsen, 1993
7 McWhirr, Viner & Wells, 1982, p.144
8 Cheek, Kate, 1998, pp.39-41
9 Spigelman, M., & Lemma E., pp.137-43
10 *ibid.*, p.143
11 Cox & Mays, 2000, p.463
12 Faerman M., Kahila, G., Smith, P., Greenblatt, C.L., Stager, L., Filon, D., Oppenheim, A., 1997, pp.212-3
13 Mays, Simon, 1993
14 Bush, H., & Zvelebil, M., 1991, p.4
15 Chamberlain, Andrew, 1994, p.14
16 Molleson, T.I., & Farwell, D.E., 1993
17 Stuart-Macadam, P., 1991
18 Hart, Gerald, 2001
19 McWhirr, Viner & Wells, p.186
20 Thomas, Lynn R., 1978
21 Bisel, Sara C., 1988, pp.61-6
22 McWhirr, Viner & Wells, pp.146 and 149
23 'A Roman Cemetery in Newarke St Leicester', dental report by Robert Carter, pp.44-9
24 Petronius, *The Satyricon*, trans. J.P .Sullivan, 1965, 33, p.55
25 Suetonius, *The Twelve Caesars*
26 Bliquez, L.J., 1996; Becker, Marshall Joseph, 1999
27 Rodwell, K.A., 1988, p.136. (I am grateful to Jean Bagnall Smith for this reference)
28 Crubézy, E., Murail, Pascal, Girard, Louis, Bernadou, Jean-Pierre, 1998. Also: Becker, Marshall Joseph, 1998
29 Wells, C., 1964, p.1
30 Lazer, Estelle, 1996, pp.620-3
31 ditto, p.621
32 Bisel, Sara C., 1987
32 *ibid.*, p.127
33 Jackson, Ralph, 1988, p.118
34 Brothwell, D.R., 1974
35 *ibid.*, p.210
36 McWhirr, Viner & Wells. p.171
37 Wakely, J., 1996
38 *ibid.*, p.40

8. PHYSICIANS AND HEALERS IN THE ROMAN WORLD

1 Nutton, 1995, p.39
2 King, 1986
3 Bowman, 1994
4 Jackson, 1988, p.86
5 King, 2001, p.39
6 trans. Michael Vickers
7 Jackson, 1993, p.81
8 *ibid.*, p.82; Nutton, 1995, p.46
9 For example, Galen I.83K; X5 and 19K, refs., cited in Jackson, 1993, p.82
10 For a cogent discussion of dates see Nutton, 2004, p.167

11 Scarborough, 1969, p.39. The concept of atoms as 'massy particles' was put on a firm basis of scientific experiment, as opposed to speculation, by a self-taught Manchester Quaker, John Dalton, who presented his Atomic Theory to the Manchester Literary and Philosophical Society in 1803. This became the foundation of modern chemistry

12 Drabkin, 1951, p.505

13 Jackson, 1988, p.56

14 Porter, 1997, p.70

15 Flemming, 2000, pp.86-7

16 Temkin, 1956, *Introduction*, p.xxxii

17 King, 1998, p.35

18 *ibid.*, pp.27-9

19 *ibid.*, p.207

20 Temkin, xli

21 Hopkins, 1966; Dickison, 1976; Riddle, 1992

22 Drabkin, 1952, p.507

23 *ibid.*, p.508

24 *ibid.*, p.509

25 Davies, 1970a, p.214.

26 Allason-Jones, 1993, p.84

27 Allason-Jones, 1993, p.1

28 Jackson, 1993, p.84

29 Boon, 1983, p.7, fn.36

30 Birley, 1972, p.89

31 Nutton, 1968

32 Webster, 1985, p.259

33 Boon, 1983, p.7 fn.36

34 King, 2001, p.38

35 Flemming, 2000, pp.256-60; Nutton, 2004

36 *ibid.*, p.258

37 *ibid.*, p.262

38 Jackson, 1988, p.61

39 King, 2001, p.42

40 Singer, 1997, pp.vii and x

41 Kiple 1997, pp.26-31

42 Gildas in Winterbottom, 108, pp.1-2

43 Nash-Williams, 1950, p.90, No. 92, fig.75 for inscription

44 I am grateful to Martin Henig for supplying these late Roman/early Christian texts

45 Salares, 2004: 'The spread of malaria in antiquity: new approaches to old problems.'

46 Kiple, pp.24 and 97

47 Plowman, R., Graves, N., Griffin, M., Roberts, J., Swan, A., Cookson, B. and Taylor, L., 1994-95, 'The Socio-economic Burden of Hospital Acquired Infection'. Public Health Laboratory Service

BIBLIOGRAPHY OF PRIMARY TEXTS

In this bibliography of primary texts, works that are readily
available in English have been used.

Aelian, *On the Characteristics of Animals*, trans. A.F. Schofield, 1959, LCL, Harvard University Press

Aeschylus, *Prometheus Bound*, trans. Philip Vellacott, 1961, Penguin Books, London

Cato, Marcus Porcius, *On Agriculture*, trans. W.D. Hooper, revised by H.B. Ash, 1967, LCL, London

Celsus, *De Medicina*, trans. W.G. Spencer, 3 vols, LCL, Harvard University Press, Cambridge, Massachusetts, and Heinemann, London. Vol.I first printed 1935, reprinted 1940, 1960. Vol.II first printed 1935, reprinted 1953. Vol.III first printed 1938, reprinted 1953, 1961

Frontinus, *The Strategems and the Aqueducts of Rome*, trans. Charles E. Bennett, 1925, (ed.) Mary B. McElwain, Heinemann, London

Galen, *Selected Works*, trans., Singer, P.N., 1997, World's Classics, Oxford University Press, Oxford

Gildas, *De Excidio Britonum*, published in 'The Ruin of Britain and Other Works', (ed.) and trans. Michael Winterbottom (Phillimore & Co., Chichester 1978) as a vol. in John Morris's *History from the Sources* series

Herodotus, *The Histories*, trans. Aubrey de Sélincourt, 1954, Penguin Books, London

Hesiod, *Theogony & Works and Days*, trans. M.L.West, 1988, World's Classics, Oxford University Press, Oxford

Hippocrates, *Hippocratic Writings*, (ed.) G.E.R. Lloyd, trans. J. Chadwick & W.N. Mann, I.M. Lonie, E.T. Withington, 1978, Penguin Books, London

Homer, *Iliad*, trans. R. Lattimore, 1951, University of Chicago Press, Ltd., London

—, *Odyssey*, trans. R. Lattimore, 1965, Harper Collins, New York, USA

Horace, *Satires and Epistles*, trans. Niall Rudd, 1979, Penguin Books, London

St Jerome, Select Letters of, trans. F.A. Wright, 1933, reprinted 1991. LBC, Harvard University Press, London

Lucian, *Satirical Sketches*, trans. Paul Turner, 1961, Penguin Books, London

Martial, *The Epigrams*, Selected and trans. by James Michie, 1978, Penguin Books, London

Ovid, *Fasti V* (Bks I-VI), trans. Sir James George Frazer, 1931, Second edition, revised by G.P. Gould, 1987, *LC*

Pausanias, *Guide to Greece*, Vols 1 and 2. trans. Peter Levi, 1971, Penguin Books, London

Petronius, *The Satyricon*, trans. J.P. Sullivan, 1986, Penguin Books, London

Plato, *Laches* and *Charmides*, trans. Rosamond Kent Sprague, 1973, Hackett Publishing Company, Indianapolis/Cambridge

—, *The Republic*, trans. Desmond Lee, 1955, Penguin Books, London

—, *Phaedo*, trans. Hugh Tredennick, 1969, Penguin Books, London

—, *Timaeus*, trans. H.D.P. Lee, 1965, Penguin Books, London

Pliny the Elder, *Natural History*, trans., H. Rackham, W.H.S. Jones & D.E. Eichholz, LCL, 1942-63, 10 vols, London

Procopius, *History of the Wars*, Books 1-11, trans. H.B. Dewing, 1914, *LCL*, Harvard University Press, London, , reprinted in 2001

Soranus, *Soranus' Gynaecology*, trans. Owsei Temkin, 1956; John Hopkins, (ed.), 1991

Suetonius, *The Twelve Caesars*, trans. Robert Graves, 1957, revised edition, with an introduction by Michael Grant, 1979, Penguin Books, Aylesbury, Bucks

Thucydides, *History of the Peloponnesian War*, trans. Rex Warner, 1954, Penguin Books, London

Varro, Marcus Terentius, *On Agriculture*, trans. W.D. Hooper, revised by H.B. Ash, 1967, LCL, London

Vitruvius, *The Ten Books on Architecture*, trans. Morris Hicky Morgan, with illustrations and original designs prepared under the direction of Herbert Langford Warren. Dover Publications, New York, 1914

BIBLIOGRAPHY OF SECONDARY TEXTS

Addyman, P.V., 1989, 'The Archaeology of public health at York, England'. *World Archaeology*, Vol.21, No.2, *Archaeology of Public Health*. Routledge, London

Allason-Jones, Lindsay, Atkinson, John & Coleman-Smith, Richard, 1979, 'Two unrecognised Roman Surgical Instruments'. *Arch. Aeliana*, Museum Notes

Allason-Jones, Lindsay, & McKay, Bruce, 1985, *Coventina's Well, A Shrine on Hadrian's Wall*, Oxbow Books, Oxford

Allason-Jones, Lindsay, & Bishop, M.C., 1988, 'Excavations at Roman Corbridge: The Hoard', *HBMC. Archaeological Report No.7*

Allason-Jones, Lindsay, 1993, 'Health care in the Roman North'. *Medicine in Northumbria*, (eds) Gardiner-Medwin, Hargreaves & Lazenby. Essays on the History of Medicine in the North-East of England, The Pybus Society, at Newcastle-Upon-Tyne

Allason-Jones, 1999, 'Health care in the Roman North'. *Britannia*, Vol.XXX

Arnott, Robert, 1996, 'Healing and Medicine in the Aegean Bronze Age'. *Journal of the Royal Society of Medicine*, Historical Reviews, Vol.89, May 1996

Aronson, J.K., 1994, *Plants in the Green College Medicinal and Herb Garden*. Pamphlet available from Green College, Oxford

Baggieri, Gaspare, 'Etruscan Wombs'. *The Lancet*, Vol.352, No.9130, 5th September, 1998, p.790

Bagnall Smith, J., 1995, 'Interim report on the Votive Material from Romano-Celtic Temple Sites'. *Oxoniensia*, LX, pp.177-205

Baker, Patricia A., 1999, 'Soranus and the Pompeii Speculum: the sociology of gynaecology and Roman perceptions of the female body'. In Baker, Forcey & Witcher (eds) *TRAC 98, Proceedings of the Eighth Annual Theoretical Roman Archaeology Conference*, Leicester 1998. Oxbow Books, Oxford, pp.141-150

Baker, Patricia A., 2001, 'Medicine, Culture and Military Identity', *TRAC 2000*, Proceedings of the Tenth Annual Theoretical Roman Archaeology Conference, held at the Institute of Archaeology, University College London, 6-8 April 2000; (eds) Gwyn Davies, Andrew Gardner & Chris Lockyear. Oxbow Books, Oxford

Baker, Patricia A., 2002. *The Roman Military Valetudinaria: fact or fiction?* pp.1-28; Medical care for the Roman Army on the Rhine, Danube and British Frontiers in the first, second and early third centuries AD. Unpublished PhD thesis. Chapter 6, 'Questioning the identification of the *valetudinaria*', pp.180-236

Baker, Patricia A., 'Taboo, Pollution and Magic: Cultural Concepts and Variations in Attitudes towards Roman-style Medical Tools,' unpublished lecture given at Reading University, 2002

Baker, Patricia A., & Carr, Gillian (eds), 2002, *Practitioners, Practices and Patients. New Approaches to Medical Archaeology and Anthropology*. Oxford, Oxbow Books

Baker, Patricia A., 'Roman Instruments: Archaeological Interpretations of their Possible "Non-Functional" Uses', *Social History of Medicine* Vol.17, No.1, pp.3-21

Ballér, Piroska, 1992, 'Medical Thinking of the Educated Class in the Roman Empire: Letters and Writings of Plutarch, Fronto, and Aelius Aristides'. In *From Epidaurus to Salerno*, Symposium held in Ravello April 1990, (ed.) Antje Krug, *PACT 34*, pp.21-24, Belgium

Barker, Philip, 1997, *The Baths Basilica, Wroxeter Excavations 1966-90*, English Heritage, Archaeological Report 8

Barnes, Henry, 1914, 'On Roman and Medical Inscriptions found in Britain'. *Proc. RSM* (section on the history of medicine), London

Bartlett, Richard, 1990, 'Latton, Harlow Temple'. In *Essex Archaeology and History* XXI, 1989

Barton, Carlin A., 1993, *The Sorrows of the Ancient Romans*, Princeton University Press, Princeton

Beagon, Mary, 1992, 'Roman Nature: The Thought of Pliny the Elder'. Chapter VI, *Ars Medicinae: Man's Use of Nature in Medicine*. pp.202-239, Clarendon Press, Oxford

Beaumann, Hellmut, 1993, *Greek Wild Flowers and plant lore in ancient Greece*, trans. and augmented by William T. Stearn & Eldwyth Ruth Stearn, The Herbert Press Ltd., London

Becker, Marshall Joseph, 1999, 'Etruscan Gold Dental Appliances: Three Newly 'Discovered' Examples'. *American Journal of Archaeology*, Vol.103, 1999, pp.103-111. *Journal of the Archaeological Institute of America*

Bellamy, David & Pfister, Andrea, 1992, *World Medicine: plants, patients and people*. Blackwell, Oxford, UK, and Cambridge, USA

Birley, Anthony, 1979, *The People of Roman Britain*. Batsford, London

Birley, Anthony, 1981, *The Fasti of Roman Britain*. Clarendon Press, Oxford

Bisel, Sara C., 1987, 'Human Bones in Herculaneum'. *Rivista Di Studi Pompeiani 1*, pp.123-129

Bisel, Sara C., 1988, 'Nutrition in First Century Herculaneum'. *Anthroplogie*, XXV1/1 1988

Bishop, M.C., & Dore, J.N., 1988, 'Corbridge: Excavations of the Roman Fort and Town, 1947-1980', *HBMC* Archaeological Report No.8, London

Blagg, T.F.C., 1986, 'The Cult and Sanctuary of Diana Nemorensis'. Pp.211-21. *Pagan Gods and Shrines of the Roman Empire*, (eds) Martin Henig & Anthony King, Oxford University Committee for Archaeology, Monograph No.8 1986

Bliquez, L.J., 1992, 'The Hercules Motif on Graeco-Roman Tools'. In *From Epidaurus to Salerno*, Symposium held in Ravello, April 1990, (ed.) Antje Krug, *PACT 34*: pp.36-50, Belgium

Bliquez, L.J., 1996, 'Prosthetics in Classical Antiquity' in *ANRW* II, 37, 3: 2640-76

Bliquez, L.J., 2003, 'Roman surgical spoon-probes and their ancient names', pp.322-30, *JRA*, Vol.16, 2003

Bloch, H., 'Aqua Traiana', *American Journal of Archaeology* 48, 1944, 337-41

Bonser, Wilfred, 1964, *A Romano-British Bibliography (AD 55-AD 449)*. Blackwell, Oxford, Vol.1 and Vol.11, (Indexes)

Boon, George, 1972. *Isca*, National Museum of Wales

Boon, George, 1974, *Silchester: The Roman Town of Calleva*. David & Charles, London

Boon, George, 1983, 'Potters, Oculists and Eye-Troubles'. *Britannia*, Vol.XIV. pp.1-12.

Boon, George, 1987, *The Legionary Fortress of Caerleon-Isca*. National Museum of Wales

Boon, George, 1989, 'A Roman Sculpture rehabilitated: the Pagan's Hill Dog'. *Britannia*, Vol.XX, pp.201-17

Bowman, Alan K., 1994, *Life and Letters on the Roman Frontier: Vindolanda and its People*. British Museum Press

Bowman, Alan K., & Thomas, David J., 1991, *The Vindolanda Writing Tablets II*, British Museum Press, London

Bowman, Alan K. & Thomas, J. David, 1994, *The Vindolanda Writing Tablets III*, British Museum Press, London

Bown, Demi, 1995, *The Royal Horticultural Society Encyclopedia of Herbs and their Uses*. BCA, London

Breeze, David J., & Dobson, Brian, 1976, revised reprint, 1987, *Hadrian's Wall*. Penguin Books,

Hamondsworth

Breeze, David J., 1994, *Roman Forts in Britain*. Shire Archaeology, Princes Risborough

Brothwell, D.R., 1974, 'Osteological Evidence of the Use of a Surgical Modiolus in a Romano-British Population: An Aspect of Primitive Technology'. *Journal of Archaeological Science*, 1974, 1, pp.209-211

Brown, Keri, in Cox, M. & Mays, S., 2000, Chapter 27 in *Human Osteology in Archaeology and Forensic Science*, published in *GMM*

Bush, H., & Zvelebil, M., 1991, *Pathology and Health in Past Societies*. BAR Int. Series 567

Chamberlain, Andrew, 1994, *Interpreting the past: Human Remains*. British Museum Press, Bloomsbury, London

Charlesworth, Dorothy, 1976, 'The Hospital, Housesteads'. *Archaeologia Aeliana*, 5th Series, Vol.4, IV, pp.17-30

Cheek, Kate, 1998, 'A Case of Spina-Bifida in Roman Britain?' *Kent Archaeological Review*, 132, pp.39-41

Ciaraldi, Marina, 2000, 'Drug preparation in evidence? An unusual plant and bone assemblage from the Pompeian countryside, Italy'. *Vegetation History and Archaeobotany*. Springer-Verlag 2000

Ciaraldi, Marina, 2002, 'The Interpretation of Medicinal Plants in the Archaeological Context: Some Case-Studies from Pompeii', (ed.) Robert Arnott, in 'The Archaeology of Medicine. Papers given at a session of the annual conference of the Theoretical Archaeology Group held at the University of Birmingham on 20 December 1998'

Collingwood, R.G., & Richmond, I., 1930, revised in 1969, *The Archaeology of Roman Britain*. Methuen & Co. Ltd, London

Collingwood, R.G., & Wright, R.P., *The Roman Inscriptions of Britain*, Vol.I., 1965, Clarendon Press, Oxford.

– Epigraphic Indexes, 1983, Goodburn, Roger & Waugh, Helen. Sutton Publishing, Stroud

Collingwood, R.G., & Wright, R.P., *The Roman Inscriptions of Britain*, Vol.II. (All published by Haverfield Bequest, Oxford)

– Fascicule 1, 1990 (eds), Frere, S.S., Roxon, M., & Tomlin, R.S.O. (*RIB* 2401-2411)

– Fascicule 3, 1991 (eds), Frere, S.S., & Tomlin, R.S.O. (*RIB* 2421-2441)

– Fascicule 4, 1992 (eds), Frere, S.S., & Tomlin, R.S.O. (*RIB* 2442-2480). Oxford

– Fascicule 6, 1994 (eds), Frere, S.S., & Tomlin, R.S.O. (*RIB* 2492-2500). Sutton
Indexes to *RIB* 11, Frere, S.S.

Corpus of Sculpture of the Roman World. Vol.1, British Academy and Oxford University Press, Oxford

– Fascicule 1, 1977, Phillips, E.J.

– Fascicule 2, 1982, Cunliffe, B.W., & Fulford, M.G.

– Fascicule 5, 1988, Brewer, Richard J.

– Fascicule 6, 1988, Coulston, J.C., & Phillips, E.J.

Cox, Margaret & Mays, Simon, 2000 (eds), *Human Osteology in Archaeology and Forensic Science*. GMM

Crubézy, E.; Murail, Pascal; Girard, Louis; Bernadou, Jean-Pierre, 1998, 'False teeth of the Roman World'. *Nature*, Vol.391, Jan. 1998. Also: Becker, Marshall Joseph, 1998, 'A Roman Implant re-considered' *Nature*, Vol.394, August, 1998

Crummy, Philip, 1996a, 'Your Move Doctor!' *The Colchester Archaeologist* 1996-7; No.10, 1-9, Colchester Archaeological Trust

Crummy, Philip, 1997b, 'The Stanway Burials'. *Current Archaeology*, 1997, No.153

Crummy, Philip, 1997c, *City of Victory*. Colchester Archaeological Trust

Crummy, Philip, 2002, *A preliminary account of the doctor's grave at Stanway*, Colchester, England, in *Practioners, Practices and Patients*. Baker & Carr (eds), 2002, Oxbow Books, Oxford

Cunliffe, Barry, 1988, *Greeks, Romans & Barbarians*. Batsford, London

Cunliffe, Barry, & Davenport, P., *The Temple of Sulis Minerva at Bath 1. The Site. OUCA*, Mon. No.7, Oxford

Dalrymple, William, 1998, *To the Holy Mountain*. Flamingo, London

Daniels, C.M. (ed.), 1989, *The Eleventh Pilgrimage of Hadrian's Wall*. Society of Antiquities of
   Newcastle upon Tyne

Darson, V., 1993, *Dwarfs in Ancient Egypt and Greece*. Clarendon Press, Oxon

Davies, Roy W., 1970a, 'The Roman Military Medical Service' in collected papers, 1989, (eds)
   Breeze & Maxwell, *Service in the Roman Army*. Edinburgh University Press, Edinburgh, with
   the University of Durham

Davies, Roy, 1970b, 'Some Roman Medicine'. *Medical History*, XIV, 1970, pp.101–106

Davies, Roy W., 1970c, 'A note on the Hoard of Roman Equipment buried at Corbridge'.
   Durham University Journal, 1970, pp.177–180

Delaine, Janet, 1999, 'Benefactions and Renewal: bath buildings in Roman Italy', Roman Baths
   and Bathing, proceedings of the First International Conference on Roman Baths held at Bath,
   England, 30 March–4 April 1992, (eds) J. Delaine & D.E. Johnston

De Wael, Ferdinand Joseph, 1933, 'The Sanctuary of Asklepios and Hygieia at Corinth'. *American
   Journal of Archaeology*, XXXVII, 1970, pp.417–451

Dickison, Sheila K., 1976, 'Abortion in Antiquity'. *Arethusa*, 1976, (6) pp.159–166

Dover, K., 1996, 'Classical Greek Attitudes to Illness'. *Vesalius*, II, 1, 34–38, 1996

Drabkin, I.E., 1951, 'Soranus and his System of Medicine'. *BHM*, No.6 Vol.XXV, Nov–Dec.
   1951, pp.503–518

Dunbabin, Katherine M.D., 1989, '*Baiarum Grata* Voluptas: Pleasures and Dangers of the Baths'.
   Papers of the British School at Rome. Vol.57, LVII, pp.6–49

Edelstein, Emma J., & Edelstein, Ludwig, 1945, reprinted in 1998, 'Asclepius: Collection and
   Interpretation of the Testimonies'. John Hopkins University Press, Baltimore and London

Edelstein, Ludwig, 1952, 'The Relationship of Ancient Philosophy to Medicine'. *BHM*, 1952,
   Vol.26, pp.296–316

Entralgo, Pedro Lain, 1970, *The Therapy of the Word in Classical Antiquity*, (ed.) and trans. L.J.
   Rather & John M. Sharp, Yale University Press, Newhaven and London. Chapter 3, *The
   Platonic Rationalization of the Charm*, pp.108–132

Evans, Harry B., 1994, *Water Distribution in Ancient Rome: the evidence of Frontinus*. The University
   of Michigan Press, Ann Arbour, 1997

Faerman M., Kahila, G., Smith, P., Greenblatt, C.L, Stager, L., Filon, D., Oppenheim, A., 1997,
   'DNA analysis reveals the sex of infanticide victims'. *Nature*, Vol.385, pp.212–213

Farrington, Andrew, 1999, *Roman Baths and Bathing*, Proceedings of the First International
   Conference on Roman Baths held at Bath, England, 30 March–4 April, 1992, (eds) J. Delaine
   & D.E. Johnston

Filer, Joyce M., 2002, 'Anatomy of a Mummy'. *Archaeology*, 27–29, March/April 2002

Fitzpatrick, A.P., 1991, '*Ex Radice Britanica*'. *Britannia*, Vol.XXII, 1991

Flemming, Rebecca, 2000, *Medicine and the Making of Roman Women*. Oxford University Press, Oxford

Flück, Hans, 1941, trans. J.M. Rowson, 1973, *Medicinal Plants and their Uses*. W. Foulsham & Co.
   Ltd, London

Frankfurter, David, 1961, reprinted 1998, *Religion in Roman Egypt: Assimilation and Resistance*.
   Princeton University Press, New Jersey

Freeth, Chrissie, 'Ancient Trips to the Dentist'. *British Archaeology*, 4/1999

Frere, Sheppard, 1990, 'Harlow Temple', *Britannia*, 22, 1991, pp.262.

Gask, G.E., & Todd, J., 1953, 'The origin of hospitals', in E.A. Underwood (ed.), *Science, medicine
   and history*. Oxford University Press

Gibbins, David, 1997, 'More Underwater Finds of Roman Medical Equipment'. *Antiquity*, 71,
   1997, pp.457–9

Gilliam, J.F., 1961, 'The Plague under Marcus Aurelius'. *The American Journal of Philology*, pp.73,
   225–51

Gilson, Andrew G., 1981, 'A Group of Roman Surgical and Medical Instruments from
   Corbridge'. *Sunderdruck aus dem Saalburg-Jahrbuch XXXVII-1981*, pp.5-9. Verlag Walter de
   Gruyter, Berlin, New York

Gilson, Andrew G., 1983, 'A Group of Roman Surgical and Medical Instruments from Cramond,

Scotland'. *Medizin Historisches Journal*, Gustav Fischer Verlag, Stuttgart, New York, pp.384-93

Girardon, Sheila, 1993, 'Ancient Medicine and Anatomical Votives in Italy'. *Institute of Archaeology Bulletin*, No.30. University of London, pp.29-40

Godwin, Harry, 1975, *A History of the British Flora*. Cambridge University Press, Cambridge

Gordon, Richard, 1992, 'The healing event in Graeco-Roman folk-medicine'. *Ancient Medicine in its Socio-Cultural Context*; papers read at the congress held at Leiden University, 13-15 April 1992, (eds) Ph. J. van der Eijk, H.F.J. Horstmanshoff, P.H. Schrijvers, Vol.1

Grant, Mark, 2000, *Galen on Food and Diet*. Routledge, London.

Green, Miranda J., 1976, *A Corpus of Religious Material from the Civilian areas of Roman Britain*. *BAR* British Series 24, pp.220 (now Aldhouse Green)

Green, Miranda J., 1983, *The Gods of Roman Britain*. Shire Archaeology (now Aldhouse Green)

Green, Miranda Aldhouse, 1999, 'Pilgrims in Stone', *BAR* International Series 754

Grmek, Mirko D., 1983, *Diseases in the Ancient Greek World*, trans. Mireille Muellner and Leonard Muellner, 1989. John Hopkins University Press, Baltimore and London

Hagelberg, Erika & Sykes, Bryan, 1989, 'Ancient bone DNA amplified'. *Nature*, Vol.342, November, 1989

Hamilton, J.S., 1986, 'Scribonius Largus on the Medical Profession'. *Bulletin of the History of Medicine*. John Hopkins University Press, Baltimore and London

Hamilton, J.S., 1987, 'A Further Note on the Dental Aspects of the *Compositiones* of Scribonius Largus'. *Bulletin of the History of Dentistry*, Vol.34, No.1

Harman, M., Molleson, T.I., & Price, J.L., 1981, 'Burials, bodies, and beheadings in Romano-British and Anglo-Saxon cemeteries'. *Bull. Br. Mus. Nat. Hist. Geol.* 35 (3), pp.145-88

Hart, Gerald, 1972, 'The earliest medical use of the caduceus'. *C.M.A. Journal*, Dec.9, 1972, Vol.107, pp.1107-9

Hart, Gerald, 1970, 'A Haematological Artefact from Fourth-Century Britain' reprinted from *Bulletin of the History of Medicine, Vol. XLIV*, No.1, Jan.-Feb. 1970

Hart, Gerald, 2000, '*Aesculapius: the God of medicine*'. The Royal Society of Medicine Press, London

Hart, Gerald, 2001, 'Descriptions of Blood and Blood Disorders Before the Advent of Laboratory Tests'. *British Journal of Haematology*, Historical Review. Blackwell Science Ltd, pp.115, 719-728

Henig, M., 1978, second edition, 'A Corpus of Roman Engraved Gems from British Sites'. *BAR*, British Series 8, Oxford

Henig, M., & Leahy, Kevin, 1984, 'A Bronze Bust from Ludford Magna, Lincolnshire'. *The Antiquaries Journal*, Vol. LXIV, part 1 pp.387-389

Henig, M., 1984, *Religion in Roman Britain*. Batsford, London

Henig, M., 1990, *The Content Family Collection of Ancient Cameos*, Ashmolean Museum, Oxford

Henig, M., 1996, *The Art of Roman Britain*. Batsford, London

Henig, M. and Vickers, M., 1993, *Cameos in Context. The Benjamin Zucker Lectures, 1990*, Ashmolean Museum, Oxford

Henneberg, Maciej, & Henneberg, Renata, 2002, 'Reconstructing Medical Knowledge In Ancient Pompeii From the Hard Evidence of Bone and Teeth'. *Studies on Nature Technology, and Science at the Time of Pompeii*. Soprintendenza Archeologica Di Pompeii

Holladay, A.J., & Poole, J.F.C., 1979, 'Thucydides and the Plague of Athens'. *The Classical Quarterly*, Vol.XXIX (new series) 1979, pp.282-300

Hood, Sinclair, 1978, *The Arts in Prehistoric Greece. The Pelican History of Art*. Penguin Books, Harmondsworth, Middlesex

Hope, Valerie M., & Marshall, Eireann, 2000, *Death and Disease in the Ancient City*. Routledge, London and New York

Hopkins, K., 1966, 'Contraception in the Roman Empire'. *Comparative Studies in Society and History* 8, 124-52

Howatson, M.C., 1937, second edition,1989, *The Oxford Companion to Classical Literature*. Oxford University Press, Oxford

Huxley, H.H., 1957, 'Greek Doctor & Roman Patient'. *Greece and Rome* pp.26, 132-8

JACT, Greeek Course, 1984, 'The World of Athens'. Cambridge University Press, Cambridge, UK

Jackson, R., 1986, 'A set of Roman medical instruments from Italy', *Britannia* Vol.XVII, pp.119-67

Jackson, R., 1988, *Doctors & Diseases in the Roman Empire*. British Museum Press

Jackson, R., 1990a, 'A new collyrium stamp from Cambridge'. *Britannia*, Vol.XXI, pp.275-83

Jackson, R., 1990b, 'Roman doctors and their instruments: recent research into ancient practice'. *Journal of Roman Archaeology*,Vol.3, pp.5-27

Jackson, R., 1990c, 'Waters and Spas in the Classical World'. *Medical History*, Supplement No.10. 1990, pp.1-13

Jackson, R., 1992a, 'Staphylagra, Staphylocaustes, Uvulectomy and Haemorrhoidectomy: the Roman Instruments and Operations', in *From Epidaurus to Salerno*. Symposium held at the European University Centre for Cultural Heritage, Ravello, April, 1990 (*PACT 34*, 1992), pp.167-185

Jackson, R., 1992b, 'Oculists' Stamps'. *Roman Inscriptions of Britain*, (eds) Frere & Tomlin, Vol.II, fasc.4, pp.43-62

Jackson, R., 1993, 'Roman Medicine: the practioners and their practices', in Wolfgang Haase & Hildegard Temporini (eds), *Aufstieg und Niedergang der römischen Welt* 11, 37.1, pp.79-101

Jackson, R., 1994, 'The surgical instruments in Celsus' *De Medicina*' in *Aspects Historiques, Scientifiques et Littéraires*, de l'Université de Saint-Étienne

Jackson, R., 1994b, 'The mouse, the lion and the crooked one: two enigmatic Roman handle types'. *The Antiquaries Journal*, London

Jackson, R., 1995a, 'The composition of Roman medical *instrumentaria* as an indication of medical practice: a provisional assessment', in *Ancient Medicine in its Socio-Cultural Context*, Vol. 1. Papers read at the congress held at Leiden University, April 1992, (eds) Ph. J. van der Eijk, H. Horstmanhoff & P.H. Schrivers. *Clio Medica*

Jackson, R., 1995b, 'A Roman Healer God from Sussex'. *British Museum Magazine*, pp.19-21

Jackson, R., 1996a, 'Eye medicine in the Roman Empire' in *Rise and Decline of the Roman World*, (eds) Wolfgang Haase & Hildegard Temporini, pp.2228-51

Jackson, R., 1996b, 'A New Collyrium-Stamp from Staines and some thoughts on Eye Medicine in Roman London and *Britannia*' in *Interpreting Roman London: Papers in memory of Hugh Chapman*, (eds) Bird, Hassall & Sheldon. Oxbow Monograph 58, Oxford, pp.177-87

Jackson, R., 1997a, 'Eye diseases in the Graeco-Roman World'. *British Museum Magazine Souvenir Issue*, No.28, Summer 1997, pp.23-5

Jackson, R., 1997b 'Ancient British Medical Medical Kit Found'. *Minerva*, 3-5, Vol.8, No.5. Sept.-Oct. 1997

Jackson, R., 1997c, 'An Ancient British medical kit from Stanway, Essex'. *The Lancet*, Vol.350, No.9089, pp.1471-74, November 1997

Jackson, R., 1997d, 'A Novel Roman Forceps'. *The Ashmolean* No.33, pp.15-16

Jackson, R., 2002a, 'Roman Surgery: the Evidence of the Instruments'. Papers given at a session of the annual conference of the Theoretical Archaeology Group held at the University of Birmingham on 20/12/98, (ed.) Robert Arnott

Jackson, R., 2002b, 'A Roman Doctor's House in Rimini'. British Museum Magazine, No.44, Autumn 2002

Jackson, R., 2003, 'The Domus "del chirurgo" at Rimini: an interim account of the medical assemblage'. *JRA*, Vol.16, 2003, pp.312-321

Jansen, Gemma, 1997, 'Private Toilets at Pompeii: Appearance and Operation'. *Sequence and Space in Pompeii*, (eds) Sara E. Bon & Rick Jones. Oxbow, Oxford, 1997

Johns, Catherine, 1982, *Sex or Symbol? Erotic images of Greece and Rome*. British Museum Press, London

Johns, Catherine, 1996, *The Jewellery of Roman Britain: Celtic and Roman Traditions*. UCL Press, London

Johns, C., & Potter, T., 1983, *The Thetford Treasure: Roman Jewellery and Silver*. British Museum

Publications, London

Johnson, Anne, 1983, *Roman Forts of the 1st and 2nd centuries AD in Britain and the German Provinces*. Adam & Charles Black, London

Johnston, Francis E., 1963, 'Some Observations on the Roles of Achondroplastic Dwarfs Through History'. Para Paedriatrics Section, *Clinical Paedriatrics*, Dec.1963, vol.2, No.12. B. Lippincott Co., Philadelphia, Montreal

Jouanna, Jacques, 1992, *Hippocrates*, reprinted 1999, trans. M.B. DeBoise. John Hopkins University Press, Baltimore and London

Karlin, Arno, 1995, *Plague's Progress: a Social History of Man and Disease*. Victor Gollancz, London

Kerényi, C., 1960, *Asklepios: Archetypal Image of the Physician's Existence*. Thames & Hudson, London

King, Antony C., 1994, *British and Irish Archaeology: a Bibliographical Guide*. Manchester University Press, Manchester

King, Helen, 1983, 'Bound to Bleed: Artemis and Greek Women', in A. Cameron & A. Kurt (eds), *Images of women in antiquity*. Croom Helm [Rev. edn Routledge, 1993], London, pp.109-27

King, Helen, 1986, 'Agnodike and the profession of medicine'. *Proceedings of the Cambridge Philological Society*, 212, pp.53-77

King, Helen, 1988, 'The early anodynes: pain in the ancient world', chapter 3 in R.D. Mann, *The History of the Management of Pain*. Parthenon Press, Cornforth

King, Helen, 1998, *Hippocrates' Woman, Reading the female body in Ancient Greece*. Routledge, London

King, Helen, 2001, *Greek and Roman Medicine*. Bristol Classical Press, Bristol

Kiple, Kenneth F., 1997, *Plague, Pox & Pestilence*. Weidenfeld & Nicolson, London

Klingshirn, William E., 1994, *Caesarius of Arles: The Making of a Christian Community in Late Antique Gaul*. Cambridge University Press, Cambridge, UK

Knights, B.A., Dickson, C.A., Dickson, J.H., Breeze, D.J., 1983, 'Evidence Concerning the Roman Military Diet at Bearsden, Scotland, in the second century AD'. *JAS*, 1983, 10, pp.139-52. Academic Press Inc., London, Ltd

Koenen, C., 1904, 'Beschreibung von Novaesium'. *Bonner Jahrbucher* 111/112: pp.97-242

Kohn, George C., 1995, *The Wordsworth Encyclopedia of Plague & Pestilence*. Wordsworth Reference, Hertfordshire, UK

Koloski-Ostrow, Ann Olga, 1994, 'Finding Social Meaning in the Latrines of Pompeii', *Cura Aquarum in Campania*. Proceedings of the Ninth International Congress on the History of Water Management and Hydraulic Engineering in the Mediterranean Region, Pompeii, 1-8 October 1994, (eds) Nathalie De Haan & Gemma C.M. Jansen, Leiden 1996. Babesh *Annual papers on Classical Archaeology*, Supplement 4, 1996.

Kruta,V., Frey, O., Raftery, B. and Szabo, M. (eds), 1991, *The Celts, the Origins of Europe*, Thames & Hudson, London

Künzl, E., 1982, 'Was soll die Maus auf dem chirurgischen Instrument?' *Antidoron, Festschrift Jurgen Thimm, Karlsruhe*

Künzl, E., 1983, *Medizinische Instrumente aus Sepulkralfunden der römischen Kaiserzeit*. Rheinlandverlag, Bonn

Künzl, E., 1984, 'Einige Bemerkungen zu den Herstellern der römischen medizinischen Instrumente'. In *Alba Regia* 21, p.59-65, Taf. XXIX-XXX

Künzl, E., Epigraphische Zeugnisse römischer augenärzte: Inschriften und Okulistenstempel, 468-81, in M. Feugere, E. Künzl & U. Weisser, Die Starnadeln von Montbellet (Saône-et Loire). Ein Beitrag zur antoken und islamischen Augenheilkunde, Jahr des Römisch-Germanischen Zentral Mainz, 4.6, 436-508

Künzl, E., 1991, 'The Tomb of the Warrior and Surgeon of München-Obermenzing and other archaeological evidence of Celtic medicine' in *The Celts, the Origins of Europe*. A volume published on the occasion of the exhibition *The Celts, the Origins of Europe* at the Palazzo Grassi, San Samuele 3231, Venice. March-December 1991

Lazer, Estelle, 1996, 'Revealing secrets of a lost city: an archaeologist examines skeletal remains from the ruins of Pompeii'. *MJA*. Vol.165 2/16 December 1996

le Strange, Richard, 1997, 'A History of Herbal plants'. Angus & Robertson, London

Liversidge, Joan, 1968, *Britain in the Roman Empire*. Routledge & Kegan Paul, London

Lloyd, G.E.R., 1950, (ed.) 'Hippocratic Writings', reprinted 1983, trans. J. Chadwick & W.N. Mann. (Harmondsworth), reprinted Penguin Books, 1983

Longfield-Jones, G.M., 1986, 'A Graeco-Roman Speculum in the Wellcome Museum'. *Medical History*, 1986, Vol.30, pp.81-89

Mabey, Richard, 1996, 'Flora Britannica'. Sinclair-Stevenson, printed and bound in Spain by Cayfosa Industria Grafica

Majno, G., 1975, 'The Healing Hand: Man and Wound in the Ancient World'. Harvard University Press, Cambridge, Mass.

Mann, John, 1992, reprinted 1999, *Murder, Magic and Medicine*. Oxford University Press, Oxford

Manniche, Lise, 1989, reprinted 1999, *An Ancient Egyptian Herbal*, British Museum Press, London

Martin, Roland, 1965, 'Wooden Figures from the Source of the Seine'. *Antiquity* XXXIX, 1965, pp.247-52

Mays, Simon, 1993, 'Infanticide in Roman Britain'. *Antiquity*, 67, 1993, pp.883-8

Mays, Simon, 1995, 'Killing the unwanted child'. *British Archaeology*, 48, March 1995

McWhirr, A., Viner, L., & Wells, C., 1982, *Cirencester Excavations 11. Romano-British Cemeteries at Cirencester. The Human Burials*. Published by the Cirencester Excavation Committee, Corinium Museum, Cirencester

Meadows, Ian, 1996, 'The Nene Valley, British or Mosell?' *Current Archaeology*, No.150, November 1996, pp.212-215

Megaw, R., & Megaw, V., 1989, *Celtic Art*. Thames & Hudson, London

Melas, Evi, 1970, *Temples and Sanctuaries of Ancient Greece*. Thames & Hudson, London

Miller, J., 1969, *The Spice Trade of the Roman Empire, 29 BC to AD 641*. Oxford University Press 1969, reprinted 1998, Sandpiper books

Miller, Timothy S., 1985, second edition, 1997, *The Birth of the Hospital in the Byzantine Empire*. John Hopkins University Press, Baltimore and London

Millett, M., & Graham, D., 1986, *Excavations on the Romano-British small town at Neatham, Hampshire, 1969-1979*. Hampshire Field Club Monograph 3, Sutton Publishing, Stroud

Molleson, T.I., & Farwell, D.E., 1993, *Poundbury* Vol.2, 'The Cemeteries'. Dorset, Natural History and Archaeological Society, Dorset. Monograph Series No.11, (ed.) Jo Draper

Montserrat, Dominic, 1998, 'Pilgrimage to the shrine of SS Cyrus and John at Menouthis in late antiquity'. From D. Frankfurter, *Pilgrimage and Holy Space in Late Antique Egypt*. Brill, Leiden

Montserrat, Dominic & Meskell, Lynn, 1997, 'Mortuary Archaeology and Religious Landscape at Graeco-Roman Deir El-Medina'. *Journal of Egyptian Archaeology*, Vol.83, 1998, pp.179-197

Morris, John, 1971, revised edition Browning, R., & Macready, S., 1998, *Londinium: London in the Roman Empire*. Wiedenfield & Nicholson, London

Morton, Julia, 1997, *Major Medicinal Plants, Botany, Culture and Uses*. Charles C. Thomas, Springfield, Illinois, USA

Murray, Oswyn, 1980, *Early Greece*, second edition, 1993. Fontana Press, London

Museum of London Publication, 1998, *Roman Bodies*, compiled by Alex Werner, pp.34-50

Nash-Williams, V.E., 1950, *The Early Christian Monuments of Wales*. University of Wales Press, Cardiff, pp.88 and 90; pp.89, fig.75

Nencini, Paolo, 1997, 'The Rules of Drug Taking: Wine and Poppy Derivatives in the Ancient World' I. General Introduction. Substance Use and Misuse, 32(1), pp.89-96; The rules of Drug Taking: Wine and Poppy Derivatives in the Ancient World. VI. Poppies as a Source of Food and Drug; Substance Use and Misuse, 32(6) pp.757-66; The Rules of Drug Taking: Wine and Poppy Derivatives in the Ancient World. VII. A Ritual Use of Poppy Derivatives? Substance Use and Misuse, 32(10), pp.1405-15

Nenova-Merdjanova, Rossitsa, 1999, 'Roman Bronze Vessels as part of the *instrumentum balnei*. Roman Baths and Bathing'. Proceedings of the First International Conference on Roman

Baths held at Bath, England, 30 March–4 April 1992, (eds) J. Delaine & D.E. Johnston

Nijhuis, Karin, 1995, 'Greek doctors and Roman patients: a medical anthropological approach', in *Ancient medicine in its Socio-Cultural Context*. Papers read at the congress held at Leiden University, 13-15 April 1992, (eds) Ph. J. van der Eijk, H.F.J. Horstmanshoff, P.H. Schrijvers, Vol.1

Nunn, John F., 1996, 'Ancient Egyptian Medicine'. British Museum Press, London

Nutton, V., 1968, 'A Greek Doctor at Chester'. *JCAS*, 55, 1968, pp.7-13

Nutton, V., 1969, 'Medicine and the Roman Army: a further consideration'. *Medical History*, Vol. XIII, 1969, pp. 261-70. The Wellcome Institute for the History of Medicine

Nutton, V., 1981, (ed.), *Galen: Problems and Prospects*. A collection of papers submitted at the 1979 Cambridge Conference. The Wellcome Institute for the History of Medicine

Nutton, V., 1985, 'The Drug Trade in Antiquity', *JRSM*. 78, No.2, February 1985

Nutton, V., 1995, 'Scribonius Largus, the Unknown Pharmacologist'. *Pharmaceutical Historian*, March 1995, Vol.25, pp.5-8

Nutton, V., 1995, 'Roman Medicine 250 BC-AD 200', in Nutton, V., 1996, 'Healers in the medical market place: towards a Graeco-Roman medicine'. *Medicine in Society, Historical essays*, (ed.) Andrew Wear. Cambridge University Press, Cambridge, UK

Nutton, Vivian, 2000, 'Medical thoughts on urban pollution', in Hope & Marshall. Routledge, London and New York, pp.65-74

Nutton, Vivian, 2004, *Ancient Medicine*. Routledge, Oxon

Painter, K., 1971, 'A Roman gold ex-voto from Wroxeter, Shropshire'. *The Antiquaries Journal*, LI, Part II, pp.329-31

Painter, K., *Pagan to Christian in the Fourth Century in Britain*. Lecture to Oxford Archaeological and Historical Society, Feb. 2000

Pedley, John Griffiths, 1990, *Paestum: Greeks and Romans in Southern Italy*. Thames & Hudson, London

Pellegrino, Edmund D., & Pellegrino Alice A., 1983, 'Humanism and Ethics in Roman Medicine: Translation and Commentary on a Text of Scribonius Largus'. *Literature and Medicine*, 7, 1988. John Hopkins University Press, pp.22-38

Petracos, Basil, 1995, *The Amphiareion of Oropos*. Monuments and Museums of Greece, Clio Editions, pp.20-22 Antiochus Str. Athens

Penn, R.G., 1994, *Medicine on Ancient Greek and Roman Coins*. Seaby, London

Petch, D.F., 1968, 'The Praetorium at Deva'. *JCAS*, Vol.55, 1968, 1-5

Phillips, E.D., 1958, 'Aesclepius, God of Healing'. *The Irish Journal of Medical Science*, Dublin

Pitts, Lynn F., & St Joseph, J.K., 1985, 'The Hospital', in *Inchtuthil, The Roman Legionary Fortress*, Britannia Mon., Series No.6. The Society for Roman Studies, London

Poole, J.F.C., & Holladay, A.J., 1979, 'Thucydides and the Plague of Athens', *Classical Quarterly* NS 29, pp. 282-300

Porter, Roy, 1997, *The Greatest benefit to Mankind*. Harper Collins, London

Potter, T.W., 1985, 'A Republican Healing-Sanctuary at Ponte di Nona near Rome and the Classical Tradition of Votive Medicine'. *JBAA*, 1985, pp.23-47, Pls.VI-XI

Potter, T.W., 1987, *Roman Italy*. British Museum Press, London

Potter, T.W., & Johns, Catherine, 1992, *Roman Britain*. British Museum Press, London

Putnam, Bill, 1997, *The Dorchester Roman Aqueduct*. Current Archaeology, No.154, pp.363-9

Ratief, Francois P., & Cilliers, Louise, 1998, 'The epidemic of Athens, 430-426 BC' in *SAMJ*, Vol.88, No.1, January 1998

Rawson, E.D. 1982, 'The Life and Death of Asclepiades of Bithinya', *Classical Quarterly* 32, pp.358-70

Richmond, I.A., 1938-9, 'The Agricolan Fort at Fendoch'. *Proceedings of the Society of Antiquiries of Scotland*, Vol.73, pp.110-54

Richmond, I.A., 'The Roman Army Medical Service'. *University of Durham Medical Gazette*, June 1952

Richmond, I.A., 1968, '*Hod Hill*' Vol.II. Trustees of the British Museum, London

Riddle, J. 1980, *Contraception and Abortion from the Ancient World to the Renaissance*. Harvard University Press, Cambridge, Mass.

Riddle, John M., 1985, 'Dioscorides on Pharmacy and Medicine', University of Texas Press, Austin, Texas

Roberts, C., & Manchester, K., 1883, *The Archaeology of Disease*, second edition, 1995. Sutton Publishing, Stroud

Roberts, Charlotte, 1988, 'Trauma and Treatment in the British Isles in the Historic Period: a design for multi-disciplinary research' reprinted from D.J. Ortner

Roberts, Charlotte A., 1988, 'A rare case of dwarfism from the Roman Period'. *Journal of Palaeopathology*, (ed.) L. Capasso, Vol.2, No.1, Marino Solfanelli Editore

Rodwell, K.A., 1988, 'A Roman Burial, the fourth tooth a pebble set in plaster'. *Chelmsford Archaeological Trust Research Report*, No.63, 1988, p.136

Rogers, J., & Waldron, T., 1995, *A Field Guide to Joint Disease in Archaeology*. John Wiley & Sons, England

Salares, Robert, 2002, *Malaria and Rome: a history of malaria in ancient Italy*. Oxford University Press, Oxford

Salares, Robert, 2004, 'The Spread of Malaria in Antiquity', Medical History 48, No.3, pp.311-28

Salazar, Christine F., 2000, *The Treatment of War Wounds in Graeco-Roman Antiquity*. Brill, Leiden, Boston, Koln

Sambon, Luigi, 1895, 'Donaria of Medical Interest'. *The British Medical Journal*, Vol.11 for 1895, London

Scarborough, John, 1969, *Roman Medicine*. Thames & Hudson, London

Scarborough, John, 1976, 'Celsus on human vivisectiion at ptolemaic Alexandria'. *Clio Medica* 11, pp.25-38

Scarborough, John, 1995, 'The Opium Poppy in Hellenistic and Roman Medicine'. *Drugs and Narcotics in History*, (ed.) Roy Porter & Mikulas Teich, Cambridge University Press, Cambridge, UK

Scarborough, J., & Nutton, V., 1982, 'The preface of Dioscorides *Materia Medica*: introduction, translation and commentary'. *Transactions and Studies of the College of Physicians of Philadelphia*, new series 4, pp.187-227

Scobie, Alex, 1986, 'Slums, Sanitation, and Mortality in the Roman World' *KLIO*. 68, 2, pp.399-433

Sherratt, Andrew, 1996a, *With baleful weeds and precious-juicéd flowers: Grooved Ware, Grape-cups and prehistoric pharmacognosy*. Unfinished draft

Sherratt, Andrew, 1996b, *Flying up with the souls of the dead*. British Archaeology No.15, May 1996, p.14

Shotter, David, 1996, *The Roman Frontier in Britain*. Carnegie Press, Preston

Singer, Charles, 1927, 'The Herbal in Atiquity and its Transmission to Later Ages'. *Journal of the Hellenic Society*, Vol.XLVII, pp.1-52

Singer, P.N., 1997, *Galen: Selected Works*. Worlds Classics, Oxford University Press, Oxford

Smith, Norman, 1978, 'Roman Hydraulic Technology'. *Scientific American*, 1978 (238), pp.154-61

Sparey-Green, Christopher, 1993, 'A Roman Medical Instrument from Dorchester'. *Proceedings of the Dorset Natural History and Archaeological Society*, Vol.116, 1994

Spigelman, Mark, & Lemma, Eshetu, 1993, 'The use of Polymerase Chain Reaction (PCR) to detect *Mycobacterium tuberculosisi* in Ancient Skeletons'. *IJO*. John Wiley & Sons Ltd, Chichester, England

Spivack, Betty S., 1991, 'A.C. Celsus: Roman Medicine'. *Journal of the History of Medicine and Allied Sciences*. Vol.46, 1991, pp.153-57

Stirland, Ann, & Waldron, Tony, 1990, 'The Earliest Cases of Tuberculosis in Britain'. *JAS*, 1990, Vol.17, pp.221-30

Strickland, T.J., 1981, 'Third Century Chester' in *The Roman West in the Third Century*, (eds) Anthony King & Martin Henig, BAR Int Ser 109, Oxford, pp. 415-444

Strickland, T.J., 1982, 'Chester: Excavations in the Princess Street/Hunter Street Area, 1978-1982. A first report on discoveries of the Roman Period'. *JCAS*, Vol.65, 1983

Stuart-Macadam, P., 1991, 'Anaemia in Roman Britain. Poundbury Camp'. *British Archaeological*

Reports, Int. Ser. No.567, (ed.) H. Bush & M. Zvelebil. British Archaeological Society, Oxford, pp.101-106

Takács, Sarolta, 1994, 'The Magic of Isis Replaced, or Cyril of Alexandria's Attempt at Redirecting Religious Devotion'. POIKILA BYZANTINA, 13, Dr. Rudolph Habelt GMBH, Bonn. Also Montserrat, 1988

Temkin, Owsei, 1935, 'Celsus' 'On Medicine' and the Ancient Medical Sects'. *BHM*, 1935, Vol.3, pp.249-64.

Temkin, Oswei, 1956, *Soranus' Gynaecology*. Baltimore

Temkin, Owsei, 1991, *Hippocrates in a World of Pagans and Christians*. John Hopkins University Press, Baltimore

Thaker, Christopher, 1994, 'Druids, Romans and Anglo-Saxons' in *The Genius of Gardening*, Weidenfeld & Nicholson, London

Thomas, Peter H., 1963, 'Personal Pleasures, 'Graeco-Roman Medical and Surgical Instruments, with special reference to Wales and the Border.' J. Coll. Gen. Practit., 1963, 6, pp.495-502

Thomas, Lynn R., 1978, 'The Dental Aspects of the *Compsitiones Medicamentorum* of Scribonius Largus: A Glimpse of Dental Treatment in the first century AD'. *Bull. of The History of Dentistry*. Vol.26, No.1: Official publication of American Academy of the History of Dentistry

Thompson, C.J.S., 1938, 'The Evolution and Development of Surgical Instruments'. *The British Journal of Surgery*, Vol.XXV, Nos.97-100, pp.726-734

Tomlin, R.S.O., 1988, *Tabellae Sulis, Roman Inscribed Tablets from the Sacred Spring at Bath*. OUCA Fascicule 1 of Monograph No.16

Tomlin, R.S.O., 1991, 'Fragment of a stilus writing tablet'. *Britannia*, Vol.XXII, p.299/24

Tomlin, R.S.O., 1992, ' Voices from the Sacred Spring'. *Bath History*, 4, pp.7-24

Tomlin, R.S.O., 1996, 'The West Deeping Lead Tablet'. *Britannia*, Vol.XXVII, pp.443-6

Tomlinson, R.A., 1983, *Epidauros*. Granada Publishing, London

Turner, R.C., & Scaife, R.G., 1995, *Bog Bodies: New Discoveries and New Perspectives*. British Museum Press, London

Von Staden, Heinrich, 1992, 'The Discovery of the Body: Human Dissection and Its Cultural Contexts in Ancient Greece'. *The Yale Journal of Biology and Medicine*, 65, 1992, pp.223-41

Wacher, John, 1995, *The Towns of Roman Britain*, second edition, Batsford, London

Wakely, J., 'A Roman Cemetery in Newarke Street, Leicester: The Skeletal Analysis'. The Leicestershire Archaeological and Historical Society,Transactions Vol.IXX, 1996. Published by the Society, The Guildhall, Leicester, pp.39 and 50

Waldron, T., 1995, *Palaeopathology Study Group, Institute of Archaeology, Gordon Square, London.* 'Changes in the Distribution of Osteoarthritis over Historical Time'. *International Journal of Osteology*, Vol. 5: pp.385-9

Webster, Graham, 1969, third edition, 1985, *The Roman Imperial Army*. A.C. Black, Whitstable, Kent

Webster, Graham, 1983, 'The Function of the Chedworth Roman "Villa"'. Transactions of the Bristol and Gloucestershire Archaeological Society 101, pp.189-92

Webster, Graham, 1986, *The British Celts and their Gods under Rome*. Batsford, London

Wedlake, W.J., 1982, 'Excavation of the shrine of Apollo at Nettleton, Wilts. 1956-1971'. Society of Antiquaries, London. *Research Reports, No.40*, 1982

Wells, Calvin, 1964, *Bones, Bodies and Disease*. Thames & Hudson, London. Textual permission granted (28/02/02) Thames & Hudson, London

Wells, Calvin, 1967, 'A Roman surgical instrument instrument from Norfolk'. *Antiquity* 41, pp.139-41

Wells, Calvin, 1973, 'A Palaeopathological Rarity in a Skeleton of Roman Date'. *Medical History*, Vol.XVII, 1973. The Wellcome Institute of the History of Medicine, Euston Road, London

Wells, Calvin, 1985, 'A medical interpretation of the votive terracottas'. App. to Potter, 1985, pp.41-4

Wenham, L., 1968, 'The Romano-British Cemetery at Trentholme Drive'. Yorks. *Archaeological Reports* No.5, HMSO, London

Wheeler, R.E.M., 1930, *London Museums Catalogues*, No.3, first edition, 1930, second edition, 1946, HMSO, London

Wheeler, R.E.M., & Wheeler, T.V., 1932, *Report on the excavation of the prehistoric, Roman, and post-Roman site at Lydney Park, Gloucestershire*, Oxford

Wickenden, N.P., 'A Copper-alloy Votive Bar and a Carved Bone Plaque from Chelmsford, Essex'. *Britannia* Vol. XVII, pp.348-51, London

Wilmanns, Juliane C., *Der Sanitatsdienst im Römischen Reich: Eine sozial geschicte Studie zum römischen Militarsanitatswesen nebst einer Posopographie des Sanitatpersonals*, Muedizin der Antike, Band 2, Hildesheim, Zurich, New York, Olms-Weidmann, 1995, pp.x, 314, illus. DM 68

Wilson, Roger, 1980, *Roman Forts*. Bergström & Boyle Books Ltd., London.

Woodward, Ann, & Leach, Peter, 1993, 'The Uley Shrines: Excavation of a Ritual Complex at West Hill, Uley, Glos. 1977-9'. *English Heritage*, London

GLOSSARY

Aetiology: the science of causation

Analgesic: that which relieves pain

Antihelmintic: destroying intestinal parasites

Arthropathy: a collection of joint pains

Augustus: 63 BC–AD 14, formerly Octavian, nephew of Julius Caesar. Emperor from 27 BC–AD 14. Originally a title with religious overtones, bestowed on Octavian by the Senate in 27 BC. Used later for an emperor with full executive powers. From the mid-second century there could be more than one Augustus at a time

Claudius: 10 BC–AD 54, emperor from AD 41 until his death in AD 54

Cortex: the outer structure of an organ or bone

Cribra orbitalia: sieve-like pitting in the roof of the eye-sockets, diagnostic of anaemia

Dental hypoplasia: poor development of dental enamel

Diaphysis: the shaft of a long bone and centre of ossification

Diptych: two-leaved, hinged ivories bestowed as gifts in Late Antiquity to celebrate marriage alliances and consulates

Diuretic: stimulating the flow of urine, either indirectly by keeping the patient cool by preventing sweating, or directly by means of drugs which stimulate the kidneys

Eburnation: polishing of bone at joints where destruction of the intervening cartilage allows bones to rub together

Endemic: habitually prevalent in a certain locality due to permanent local causes

Epidemic: widely prevalent but not usual

Epiphysis: the articular surface of a long bone. It is separated by cartilage from the diaphysis, from which the bone grows

Epode: a charm or incantation

Etruscans: A pre-Roman people of central Italy, and in early times Rome's principal rivals for the control of that area

Frontinus, Sextus Julius: c.AD 30–c.104

Gaius Caesar: 'Caligula', AD 12–41, emperor from AD 37–41

Haemolytic: that which breaks up blood cells

Lucian: c.AD 115–after 180. A satirist who scathingly, if humorously, indicts the follies of his day. He was born at Samosata, on the Euphrates in Syria; the author of some eighty prose pieces in various forms

Macroscopic: may be seen with the naked eye

Marcus Aurelius: AD 121–80, Roman emperor from 161 to his death. He shared the throne with Lucius Verus. His twelve books of 'Meditations' were written in Greek during the last ten years of his reign, whilst he was on campaign. His reign was dominated by warfare against invaders on all fronts

Metu: plural of *met*, Egyptian = vessels; the word has no direct connection in English

Microscopic: may only be seen with a microscope

Narcotic: inducing sleep, large doses can be fatal

Nymphaeum: a shrine of the nymphs; the term is used more widely to denote any building associated with a fountain, particularly one with elaborate architectural and sculptural decorations

Opus quadratum: squared stone masonry, ashlar (masonry of rectangular blocks dressed to a vertical face)

Pandemic: prevalent over the whole of the country or continent, or over the whole world

Pericles: c.495-429 BC. Athenian statesman, a professed Democrat. The funeral oration which was delivered over the Athenian dead after the first year of the war with Sparta expresses his high concept of Athens and Athenian democracy. Greatly admired by the historian Thucydides

Pharmaka: medicaments applied internally or externally

Pneuma: hot air integrated into the functioning of the body

Porotic hyperostosis: soft and porous bones

Principate: the early Empire, when the Emperor was just *principes*, first citizen

Rhizotomos: root-cutter, supplier and applier of medical materials

Sacro-iliac: the joint, or auricular surface between the sacrum and the ilium

Scurvy: a condition resulting from lack of vitamin C, ascorbic acid, in the diet; i.e. fresh fruit and vegetables

Sibylline books: the prophetic works housed in the temple of Jupiter on the Capitol at Rome

Sophrosyne: modesty, sense, prudence, discretion, chastity

Sophocles: c.496-406 BC. One of the greatest Athenian tragedians, also a musician. His early life coincided with the expansion of the Athenian Empire; he was twice elected *strategos* (general). When the cult of Asclepius was introduced into Athens he received the sacred snake representing the god in his house until the temple was ready, and composed a paean in his honour

Spina-bifida occulta: incomplete ossification of vertebrae leaving the posterior spinal membrane and cord partially exposed. There may be varying degrees of nerve function

Spondylitis: inflammation of the joints between the vertebrae

Suture: in surgery, a stitch; or a junction between two bony surfaces

Symphysis: a point of junction; usually applied to paired bones, such as the mandible and the pubic bone

Techne: art, a body of knowledge in combination with a set of skills

Torus: a smooth bony growth occurring in the frontal, mandible, maxilla or occipital bones

Trabecular disruption: damage to the internal stress-bearing network of the bone

Trauma: injury with pain

Unguentarium: a glass or pottery vessel for the containment of ointment or oil, usually taken to the baths

Vermifuge: expelling intestinal worms

Zoonoses: diseases with a primary animal host but transmissible to human beings

INDEX

If you are interested in purchasing
other books published by The History Press, or in case you have
difficulty finding any of our books in your local bookshop,
you can also place orders directly through our website

www.thehistorypress.co.uk